THE DEAD BEDROOM FIX

BY D.S.O.

www.dadstartingover.com

Who This Book is For

This book was written for heterosexual men in long-term monogamous relationships who want more sex.

Yes, I realize that there is a growing phenomenon of women being frustrated with their own lackluster sex lives. Sorry, ladies. This book is not for you.

If you are a woman and your libido is outpacing your husband/boyfriend, I can save you a lot of time and money and give you some quick solutions to try out:

1. **Concentrate on making yourself look young and pretty.** Yes, it's shallow and stupid. We're talking about MEN here. There is a reason why I listed this first. Don't overthink things. Men are visual creatures. Just look at porn, strip clubs, your husband's eyes as that young pretty gal walks by him, etc. Yes, the shallow stuff matters. A lot.

2. **Don't be a controlling asshole.** Nothing is more of a turnoff than a nagging, emasculating woman. Try empathy and sweetness, instead. Give up control and let him take over every now and then. Yes, he will make mistakes. This is not a big deal. Don't freak out on him and shame him for trying to help and trying to be a better man. The net positive return from you giving up control is far greater than the negative impact of a few silly mistakes on his part.

Loosen up. Go with the flow. Enjoy life. Enjoy your

husband. Be a cool sexy chick. Submissiveness and joy are attractive.

Encourage him. I know he annoys the shit out of you half the time and you've lost a great deal of respect for him over the years, but he's your man and you want more sex, right?

3. **Is he watching and masturbating to porn on a regular basis?** Unfortunately, excessive consumption of porn can be addictive. It can drain him of his energy and have profoundly negative effects on his well-being and behavior. Want to be different and sexy? Watch porn with him. Make it a dirty thing you two do together as a couple. Tell him what you like. Tell him YOU want to be his porn star.

4. **None of the above issues apply to your situation?** Tell him to get his testosterone checked. Yes, seriously. It's not natural for a dude to turn down sex repeatedly. He should want it frequently. Something is up and it MIGHT be that his hormones are out of balance and he needs a simple tune up. Many women report that they "got their husband back" after he started a regimen of Testosterone Replacement Therapy.

There's your dead bedroom fix, ladies. If these don't work, it's time to move on. You're a woman. Let's be honest... you could get sex this afternoon if you wanted to. Seriously. It's a totally different ballgame for men.

Now, kindly go away. Us men need to chat about you behind your back. You are WAY more complicated than we are and this will take an entire book to break down.

Before We Get Started...

Let's get some important things out of the way.

1. **I'm going to assume your wife is healthy.** It may seem obvious to most of you, but I have heard more than a few times:

"Well, it all started when my wife was diagnosed with breast cancer..."

"She suffers from depression and was recently put on meds. Since then, she has no libido."

"We had a baby one month ago. It was a very rough pregnancy. Cesarean. We almost lost the baby. Now she has zero interest in sex."

Give the woman a break! The poor thing is a human being. Those are big roadblocks in the way of her sexual desire. Give her time and have some empathy. Be a partner to her. Get her the help that she needs.

In sickness and in health, remember?

2. **I'm going to assume that YOU are healthy.** If you have issues that impact your day-today life (chronic disease, hormonal issues, mental health issues, etc), then your situation is officially above my pay grade. Get those issues ironed out and then come back to this book. You have bigger fish to fry, my friend.

3. **You need to set aside your preconceptions of what causes sexual desire in your wife.** You need to set aside your notions of what she SHOULD do as your wife and partner. You need to set aside these crippling thoughts about what you DESERVE as her man. What you've done so far is flat out not working, so it's time for plan B.

Stop reading stories online from men talking about their all-too-common "low libido" and "asexual" wives and "that's just how marriage is". Ninety percent of the time those stories are from men who just don't get it. They will never get it. Don't become part of the long line of men trying like hell to join the growing **"I AM A HELPLESS VICTIM"** parade. Stay away from these people. Their mindset is poisonous.

4. **You may be offended by what you read in this book.** Some of the things I say may seem a bit "out there". It may even seem offensive. Sexist. Bone-headed. Antiquated. Misogynistic.

Fine, I get it. Really, I do. I was in your shoes years ago and would've laughed at a book like this back then. I was way too "smart" and "educated". I knew better. Hindsight is 20/20, of course.

All I can tell you is that this WORKS. Feelings be damned… You need solutions. From my experience, what I outline in this book is the best and most direct path to getting the sex you need.

4

My Story

I'm a 40-something divorced dad of three kids. I care for my kids four days a week.

I work full-time (plus the world of dadstartingover.com), cook, clean, fold clothes, help with homework, play, discipline, chauffer, counsel, etc.

I have basically played the role of both mom and dad for years.

This is not exactly "fun". It certainly isn't easy. It's most certainly not the life I planned for. Not by a long shot.

It's fucking exhausting.

Before becoming divorced dad extraordinaire, I endured a 15-year marriage that could be described as, "roommates who once in a blue moon had sex that resulted in babies". She was just one very fertile woman and I was one very fertile dude. Don't let my three kids convince you that our sex life was abundant. It wasn't. At all. It was, by definition, a very "dead bedroom".

My ex-wife: *"I don't know why I don't feel like having sex. I just don't."*

To make a very long and very painful story short, fifteen years into our marriage (and twenty years as a couple) she was caught in a physical affair with another man. I regrettably found out ALL of the dirty little details (thank you, mobile phone technology). Yes, I caught the affair early on, but my "low libido" wife was still more than able to muster up enough energy to get a WHOLE LOT of crazy sex done in those few short months.

After I saw the evidence of the affair and all of the dirty details, I said what every man in my position says:

"She did THAT with HIM? She would never do THAT with ME?!"

I endured years of almost zero intimacy during our marriage. I thought the kind of closeness, affection and filthy sex I craved only happened in movies. I was very wrong. The real-life porn movie was happening alright… but my character didn't have a role in the sexy scenes. My scenes involved changing diapers and mowing the lawn.

I felt cheated. I felt like a dumb schmuck that was taken advantage of. I was hurt, angry and confused. My entire world was turned upside down. My past, my current life, and my future were all called into question with one horrible act by my wife.

I experienced very real depression or the first time in my life.

Looking back on my early childhood, I never saw true romance or lustfulness with my parents. I didn't see it with my friends' parents, either. Later in life, I didn't see it with most of my adult friends and their marriages.

Everyone just acted like roommates with kids. Two boring people going through the motions and running the family machine.

I just figured this was the way marriage was. Boring, but necessary. It's something we all go through in life, right? We learn that we need to temper our expectations and be grateful for what we have. Not everything has to be wine and roses. Sometimes you must ENDURE hardship for the greater good of the family and community. Just because you WANT something doesn't mean you get it. That's how life works.

Then I found out that my wife DID want the same things out of life. She wanted the same exciting relationship and the same level of sexuality and eroticism that I always wanted.. She just didn't want that with me.

Ouch.

She filed for divorce immediately after the affair was discovered. It was the best thing to ever happen to me.

I don't know what got into me, but after a brief trip down the well of depression, I went on one hell of a self-improvement kick. I just couldn't let this awful experience destroy me. I had three little ones looking up to me as their oasis of normalcy. Their mom was acting very strange and erratic. She spent less time with the kids as the months and years went by.

I've learned a lot about myself over these post-divorce years. I've learned I need a mission to keep my engine going. A purpose. I thrive on activity and can easily slip into lulls and use my busy home and work life as an excuse for laziness. Discovering the affair and the subsequent divorce were exactly the fuel I needed to get my engine going again.

I quickly learned that there are A LOT of guys out there just like me. I read a lot about the phenomenon and eventually I write a lot about the topic, too (an old hobby of mine). It's therapeutic.

I start a website at **dadstartingover.com**. I get some hits. I get a few emails. I help out a few men here and there with their issues. I seem to have tapped into something.

The most popular topics on my website, by far, are those related to "Dead Bedrooms" and cheating wives. Men just aren't getting the sex they want, and they want to fix it. They NEED to fix it... and many come to my site after it's already too late.

I decided to write this book not just to capitalize on the popularity of the topic, but to also get to the bottom of a common issue that can and will grow into something more insidious if it's not resolved early on.

Half of all marriages end in divorce. It's a common statistic we're all familiar with. It's an even higher rate of divorce for second marriages. What you may not know is that women initiate 70% of the divorces… 80% if the woman is college-educated.

Women, in general, are not happy within the confines of a typical marriage. Dead bedrooms and cheating wives reflect this.

Yes, I Married Again.

So, what's different this time around? Anything?

Oooooh yeah, it's different, alright.

We have lots of amazing sex. We have intimacy. We have romance. We love each other a great deal. We are what you would call a "nauseating" couple. We have been this way, consistently, for almost eight years.

This is my life now. There is no alternative. If the sex life and intimacy go bye-bye, so does my commitment as her husband and partner and we are no longer married.

Wow, that sounds really cold and blunt, doesn't it?

I'm cold and blunt because I know that without physical intimacy, there is no need for a monogamous relationship. None. I can get a roommate anywhere. I have friends. I can make more friends. I can get girlfriends. I can get meaningless sex. Been there, done that. It's not what I want out of life, but it's always an option.

The logistics, friendship and comfortability of our life together doesn't negate the need for real physical intimacy. You will never hear me say, "The relationship is perfect... except for the sex."

No sex = no relationship.

Don't misinterpret this as me saying, *"She better give me sex, or else!"* That's not at all what I'm saying. I'm saying that a lack of sex in a romantic relationship is indicative of much deeper issues that proliferate beyond the bedroom. As the author of this book, I know what it takes to "keep the spark alive" in my relationship. If my wife takes in all I have to offer and her response is, "Yeah… great. I still don't want you", then I know we are done.

Simply put, not having sex is a sign of a broken marriage.

You may still be a married couple, but you're no longer in a romantic relationship.

I'm looking for something special in the woman I call "wife". I'm looking for a true partner. I want somebody to experience wonderful and not-so-wonderful things with during my 80+ orbits around the sun. A good chunk of this life of mine revolves around sex. I don't hide this fact. I'm a dude, after all. I have the genitals to prove it.

So far, our intimacy is off the charts. I have volumes of dirty photos and videos that my WIFE has sent me over the years. We have a very sexy/kinky side to our lives that nobody else knows about. That is our little secret. To our friends, we are just a very sweet and loving couple that hug and smooch a lot.

In my first marriage, I was a frequent "user" of porn, if you know what I mean. In my current marriage, porn is not a thing for ME to use as a coping mechanism, but rather a sexy tool that we view together. She enjoys doing these "dirty" things together as a couple. This is part of the secret, fun and sexy side of our relationship that keeps us bonded together.

She has a body that most women at any age would kill for. She has a naturally good shape, but she also works hard to keep it looking nice. I let her know I appreciate how sexy she is by banging the snot out of her, cuddling with her for hours and showering her with praise and affection.

We are in a constant battle of keeping in shape for each other. Yes, we sometimes let life get in the way and our sexiness slips a little here and there. With my genetics, I can put on ten pounds just by looking at a piece of cake. She then cranks up the yoga and cardio, sends me a sexy photo, I drool for hours… and the next day I hit the gym with just a little more oomph and lay off the carbs.

This is healthy and normal.

What about money? My wife has her own money. More than me, actually. She has a great career as an MD. She doesn't need me to pay her bills or to buy her that nice purse she really wants. She needs me for physical/emotional intimacy and love. I'm not the provider of paycheck. I provide in other ways.

I'm her rock. I'm her partner. I'm her man.

I must keep up the hard work. I must earn this quality of a

relationship. It can go away tomorrow. I don't want to sign another round of divorce papers wondering "What if…?" It's not easy, and that's the way it should be.

I am crazy about the girl. That doesn't negate my own needs. My love and devotion are not unconditional.

For me, Dead Bedroom = Dead Marriage.

I'm never doing that again.

CHAPTER 1
What is a Dead Bedroom?

"Despite my 30 years of research into the feminine soul, I have not yet been able to answer . . . the great question that has never been answered: *What does a woman want?*"

Sigmund Freud

The "Dead Bedroom" is just what it sounds like: A monogamous romantic relationship with little to no sexual activity between the two partners.

For the purposes of this book and the intended audience, we will stick with the tried and true trope of the horny husband and the cold, disinterested wife.

It's a well-known cultural meme and has been for a long, long time.

"Marriage is a lot like prison, but without the sex." – Anonymous

"Married sex is like being awake during your own autopsy. It is root canal work without anesthetic." – Al Goldstein

"I know nothing about sex, because I was always married." – Zsa Zsa Gabor

"Sex is the most beautiful thing that can take place between a happily married man and his secretary." – Barry Humphries

These stereotypes didn't just fall from the sky. The dead bedroom happens, and it happens a lot.

You've seen this dynamic played out again and again on television and in the movies. You see it with your friends and their relationships. You probably saw it with your parents.

You think back on your childhood and remember yourself as a little boy, sitting at the dinner table on Thanksgiving Day. Dad is cutting the turkey and says something about the "juicy breast" and gives your mom a playful smile and wink. You weren't quite sure what was going on, but his energy made you smile and laugh.

But then... your mom's tone changes instantly. She gives him an angry look and says "Seriously?" as she lets out a frustrated sigh and shoves another forkful of food in her face. Dad doesn't take it well. He pouts the rest of the day and ignores everyone while watching football.

The negativity in the house was palpable.

Fast forward to now and your relationship with your wife. You come home after a long day at the office. The commute was extra annoying, and you just want to put your feet up and relax... but you can't. You immediately tend to the kids, help with dinner, take out the trash, answer some work emails, help your son with homework, play tea time with your daughter and then help put everyone to bed. Finally, after 3 bedtime stories, your job is done, and it is time to relax.

You plop in bed next to your wife. She's wearing sweatpants and a stained t-shirt. Not very sexy, but you're a man and it's been a while since you last had sexual release (beyond your usual porn/masturbation sessions). You make your typical sexy growl sound that you think is so funny, playfully squint your eyes, smile, and move your hand to her breast.

She immediately grabs your hand and pushes it away.

"Seriously? Can you just give it a rest for one night?"

She rolls over and turns off the light.

You would be mad or confused if this was a new thing. Instead, you're just sad. This is normal for your marriage and has been for a while.

She says, "Give it a rest for one night", but it's been two months since you had any kind of physical intimacy.

She holds the master key to your sex life and the door is locked. It has been locked for way too long.

As a son, husband and father, the message is clear:

The man is a horny, out-of-control bag of testosterone that needs to be put in his place.

His energy must be redirected towards the more important tasks, like providing for the family, helping with chores, and letting his wife get much-needed rest. If he doesn't leave her alone, there is hell to pay.

The woman is the cold, bossy and domineering presence in the home. She keeps things on track and must occasionally swat away at his attempts to bring sexuality into their world.

"No! Bad dog!"

When dad veers off the assigned path, he must be punished and reminded of his primary and preferred role as the provider. Mom will not hesitate to say or do something that will emasculate him and make him feel like a pervert for introducing sexuality into their relationship. It's not about hurting his feelings. It's about stopping his annoying and inappropriate behavior.

As a result, dad will act like a baby for a while. He'll eventually get over it and then the process starts all over again. Rinse and repeat.

Sound familiar?

Maybe your situation isn't THIS bad, but you ARE reading this book right now which means one thing is certain: You sure aren't happy with your sex life. **This has GOT to change and the sooner the better.**

You Are Not Alone

On my website at **dadstartingover.com**, I have written dozens of articles on a variety of relationship and self-improvement topics. By far, my most popular topics are Dead Bedrooms and female infidelity. The same goes for my podcast. Any episode related to "Dead Bedrooms" is way far ahead of any other episode.

On the popular website **www.talkaboutmarriage.com**, the two most active "focused" topics are "Sex in Marriage" and "Coping With Infidelity."

On the popular website **Reddit.com**, the DeadBedrooms forum (subreddit) has over 250,000 subscribers.

People sure do seem to have issues with sex and marriage. It's not surprising, is it? Traditional marriage goes against our basic and animalistic nature. Marriage tells men, *"You know that urge you have to bang every pretty woman you see? Stop that. Here's your one woman for the rest of your life. You'll love her and want her, but she may or may not want to have sex with you... and there's really nothing you can do about it. So... Have fun!"*

At the same time, marriage tells women, *"I know you dream of finding the all-around best guy for you to settle down with and make babies. Good luck with that! You're not worthy of 'winning' such a guy, so here's some boring schmuck who is about as far from your ideal lover as you can get. But... don't worry. He will provide for you and your children and he will love you a great deal. The good news is that you don't have to have sex with him. He'll still take care of you, regardless. You'll probably end up loathing him. Enjoy!"*

Marriage doesn't have to be this way... but more often than not, it sure does go in that direction.

What Caused YOUR Dead Bedroom?

The no bullshit truth: **Your wife isn't attracted to you.**

If she was, you would know it. You wouldn't be Googling "Wife doesn't want sex" at midnight while she snores next to you in bed. Instead you would be covered in sweat and sleeping with a smile on your face.

Instead of asking, "Why am I in a dead bedroom?", you should instead ask, *"Why is my wife no longer sexually attracted to me?"* That's when you start to get down to the actual cause of your problem.

The dead bedroom is most likely the result of a series of negative actions or inactions on the part of the man. The man was presented with all the typical obstacles that get in the way of sex (kids, stress, time, familiarity, bored wife) and he didn't respond in the correct way. These actions and inactions over the years never properly pushed the buttons his wife needed pushed to activate her sex drive (especially after parenthood).

You did X and you got Y in return. It's that simple.

Yep, I just put the responsibility for this situation squarely on your shoulders. Kinda shitty and presumptuous of me, right? Yes, it is. But, there's good reason for me to come to this conclusion.

I've heard about 10,000 dead bedroom stories from men, and after much back-and-forth, soul-searching, and honest reflection, they always come to the same conclusion: He royally fucked up somewhere along the way. He either erroneously stayed with the absolute WORST partner imaginable (many men I talk to suffer from emotional and physical abuse at the hands of their wife), or he actually married a really good woman who naturally responded to her husband's mistakes in a very predictable way: **She lost attraction to him.**

Your situation could be different than everyone else. I sincerely doubt it.

The Good News is That YOU Probably Caused This, so YOU Can Probably Fix It.

You're a dude. You like to fix things, right? That's why you're reading this book. You want to find out what part of the relationship machine broke down and caused it to stop working and spill oil all over the garage floor.

Make no mistake about it, your relationship is broken.

Sex is not just one little tiny aspect of an overall awesome relationship (like many "low-libido" wives will say). It's the biggest part.

Without sex, you are just roommates.

Without sex, you are not fulfilling your most basic human need.

Without sex, you will experience a cascading series of events that will ultimately lead to a lesser version of yourself and the end of your marriage.

If the relationship is not maintained properly, it will break down. If you put the wrong kind of oil in, the motor will seize up. You'll be left on the side of the road, scratching your head and wondering what to do next.

Unfortunately, relationships don't come with an owner's

manual. We received numerous textbooks in school, but none of them titled, "How to be the kind of man your wife will want to fuck for many years."

But, for some strange reason, men all sure seem to act like this non-existent book of rules really DOES exist.

This mystery book is packed with libido-igniting nuggets of wisdom like:

1. **Buy her gifts**. Flowers. Chocolates. Massages. Make her feel appreciated.

2. **Do more chores.** Take the stress away from her life.

3. **Happy wife, happy life!** Be more agreeable. Less drama and less stress are a good thing.

4. **Pretend that no other females in the world exist.** Your focus should be solely on your wife. Temper your sexual urges.

5. **Talk to her.** Make sure she really understands the problem and sees things from your point of view. Appeal to her rational side. Open up to her, emotionally.

In theory, they all sound great. You're more giving, you're a better housekeeper, you're more agreeable, you're more open with your feelings and you're more devoted. What's not to like?

What's funny is that every one of these are the exact opposite of what men should do when the sex goes south. In fact, they are the continuation and amplification of what caused your dead bedroom in the first place.

That's right, if we want to look at the CAUSE of the dead bedroom, we just need to look at what men typically do to try and fix it. It's the same damn thing.

How ironic.

Let's look at each of the five solutions that men try again and again. Let's break down just how and why each fails so miserably… and why we continue trying anyway.

CHAPTER 2
The Common Mistakes

"For things to reveal themselves to us, we need to be ready to abandon our views about them."

Thich Nhat Hanh

Mistake #1: Gift Giving

We all know the tried-and-true stereotype of the nervous guy showing up to the first date with flowers. Maybe he takes it up a notch and adds a box of chocolates. The chocolates may be reserved for Valentine's Day, but he will for sure keep buying gifts throughout their first date. He will buy drinks. Dinner. Maybe a little stuffed teddy bear. "Awww!" she says throughout the night.

What's he saying with all this gift-giving?

"Ok, here's the deal. You just sit there and look good and I'll give you free stuff. Sound like a plan? No, I don't expect anything from you. You don't have to qualify yourself. Your vagina and the possibility of one day being inside of it is more than enough for me. Here, let me buy you something else so you don't forget how good I am."

If for some reason the flowers and constant gift-giving results in a girlfriend, then the conditioning has been imprinted in the man.

Gift-giving = Affection from women.

What if he had NOT bought things for her right up front? What if he expected her to chip in for everything or that, God forbid, SHE should pay for dinner. Would she go on a second date and eventually marry him? No, probably not. She would tell you the same thing. She liked that he was so generous. It made her feel special.

31

So, what does that tell you?

He bought her affection.

Does that bode well for long-term romantic love? Maybe…
Maybe not.

Maybe you have convinced yourself that your wife has
EARNED your gifts you regularly give to her. Even though
she doesn't seem to have any attraction towards you and
treats you like a nuisance, she IS your wife. That is, in itself,
worthy of praise, right?

Let's be honest. You're rewarding your wife for simply being
the female in the relationship. If we examine it further, it's
also a subtle form of sexism. You're putting her up on a
pedestal just because she has boobies and a hoohah.

You're being creepy.

This is the pathetic theme to your gift giving:

*"I don't get much in the way of sex… and we all know you
don't like me all that much… so I need to bribe you to keep
you around. I'll take whatever crumbs I can get. Please,
don't leave."*

Guess what? She's fully aware of the dynamic at play here.
She knows she has you by the marbles and she will drag
this relationship on as long as possible to extract as many

resources from you as she can.

This is not evil. This is human nature.

Young girls get their homework done for them and a free ride to the mall. Women get free flowers, meals, drinks, a shoulder to cry on and later… a doting husband.

What do men not get in return? **Great sex.**

More specifically, they don't get a woman who finds them sexually attractive. It never works out in the end. Ever.

What the gift-giving does is put you right away in the mode of the "Provider".

The Provider readily gives up his resources: time, money and commitment. He does so out of an instinctual male need to make sure his tribe is safe and secure… and out of the thinly-veiled hope of getting the pretty lady to have sex with him. **It's extremely NEEDY behavior.**

The Provider sees his consistent GIVING as a positive personality trait that puts him above those in the shallow Lover category (I'll cover more about the lover/provider dynamic later). He will NEVER admit that his good deeds are anything but 100% altruistic. He's doing his manly duty, after all. This is expected of him.

If he was being honest, he would admit that he gave and gave for the purposes of getting something in return.

The truth is, he just wants love and affection and giving was his way of trying to earn those rewards. When it doesn't work out, he gets pissed. When he emotes to others about his relationship problems, the first thing he brings up are the gifts he gave her.

"But…I bought her flowers last week!"
"But…I got her that bracelet last month!"
"But… I paid for that house cleaning service she wanted!"

The message from the man is clear: *"I'm a very needy guy. I NEED my wife and her affection. The understood deal between us is that I do nice things for her, and she's SUPPOSED to reward me with sex."*

Unbeknownst to the husband, what does this gift-giving subconsciously tell his wife?

"Being a cold and disinterested wife gets my husband to take action and buy stuff that I want. Yes. he's pitiful and I lost respect for him years ago, but at least I get stuff out of it. I like stuff. I better keep treating him like dirt. This is working."

Human Psych 101: **Reward a certain behavior and you'll get more of it.**

It's all about conditioning. Much like Pavlov's dog… we're easily trained animals.

The husband is conditioned to believe, from a young age, that gift-giving results in the romantic relationship he wants. This continues into adulthood and becomes a fallback "fixer" strategy for when things start to go bad.

This is an absolute no-win situation.

Gift-giving should always come from a genuine place with no ulterior motive. It should come from the mindset of rewarding somebody for being a good person. You should never expect anything in return. You do so because you love and appreciate your partner… Not because you want more blowjobs.

Do you really love and appreciate your wife when she emasculates you and shames you for still wanting her after all these years?

No.

Then why reward her? Because you hope to turn her attitude around.

By giving gifts you are simply doubling down on your provider role in an underhanded way. Your gifts are not genuine. She innately knows this.

You're being manipulative. You're being creepy. You're being needy. You're being pathetic.

Provider = Comfort and safety. Comfort does not

necessarily equal sexual attraction (more on this later).

Provider with an ulterior motive = Creepy and needy. Creepy and needy equals revulsion.

There's no way to win here. Cut it out.

Mistake #2: Doing More Chores

There is nothing special about doing chores. They must get done. Having a penis doesn't give you a "get out of doing chores" card, as many men still believe. If the sink is full of dishes, you put them in the dishwasher. If the trash is full, you take it out. You make the bed. It's not rocket science. It's not difficult. Contrary to popular belief, doing household chores is not tough. It's annoying, but it's not difficult.

Building a bridge or drilling for oil is tough. Pulling a sheet over a mattress is something a 70-year-old grandma can do.

So why do I list doing more chores as a "mistake" if I seem so adamant about doing them? Well, the problem comes when you do these much-needed household chores and proudly bring it up to mommy... err... your wife.

"Honey, I put away the dishes for you!!"

Well whoopty-fucking-doo, little man. Welcome to adulthood. Want a cookie?

No, you want love and affection. It's obvious.

It's extremely needy behavior. It's a giant turnoff.

Running a household takes work. Not all that work is manly or intellectually stimulating. Some of it are things like cleaning the cat box and folding laundry. If you see it needs to be done and you have time to do it, you do it. That's called being an adult. That's what we all do.

By bragging about it or doing it with a future reward in mind, you're lowering yourself to a sub-adult level. My youngest child used to love to show me how he cleaned up a mess (he usually just made it worse). He wanted to impress me and show me that he was a big boy now. He needed my approval.

That's precisely what you are doing. You're not getting sex, so you bump up your housework in an effort to gain approval from your wife.

You are acting like a child. You're being very needy. Your wife doesn't want to fuck a needy child. She wants a man.

She wants the kind of guy who does the annoying and time-consuming tasks and never brings it up. She wants a scenario like this:

Her: "Wait… did you fix the lamp, fold the laundry AND clean that stain on the carpet?"

You: "Ummm… yeah?"

Her: "When did you find time to do that?!"

You: "I dunno… last night, I think."

Her: "Thank you, baby!! I just noticed. That is so awesome."

You: "No problem, sweet cheeks."

That sound like a positive exchange? That sound like something an adult MAN would do? Of course. He just did the work and never mentioned it. It had to get done. He really doesn't give a shit if she approves or not. That's not the purpose of the work. The purpose of the work was to alleviate the issue of the annoying flickering lamp, the giant pile of clothes, and the carpet that had an annoying yogurt stain on it.

There were problems. He fixed them. Simple as that. No big deal. Certainly nothing you do to win sexual intimacy or attention from your wife.

Why do so many men fall back on doing additional chores to try and reignite their wife's sex drive?

Men are fixers.

Sex life broken? Well then, let's get to patching up these holes and get this sex boat floating again!

Step one: LISTEN to the wife for guidance. Does she complain? Well, yeah. Of course. She's a woman. If she's breathing, she's complaining.

What exactly is she complaining about the most?

She is very TIRED. This seems to be the overall theme to her day-to-day existence. She's constantly worn out. She's overwhelmed to the point of exhaustion. The kids. The job. The house. She will usually point to this extreme exhaustion as the primary cause for her lack of libido.

Well, you can't make the kids go away and you can't make her job at the office any easier… but you CAN do more housework for her! That's it, then. That's the new fixer strategy. Do more housework. Yes, this is genius.

When she comes home, you will point out that you did the dishes, folded the laundry and cleaned the cat litter box. She will jump for joy, collapse into your arms and then promptly rip her clothes off and rediscover that sex drive of hers that went missing for so long… right?!

Yeah, no. It doesn't work.

See… again… you're doing things because you want to get something out of it. You can try to convince yourself that you're just being a good partner, but we both know that's bullshit.

If your wife sat you down and said, "Honey… look, no matter what you do or say, we are never having sex again. Ever. EVER.", you would be camped out in the garage pouting all day. Chores wouldn't even be on the radar.

You're doing things for mommy's approval. It's obvious. It's needy. It's weak.

Chores are like taking a shit. It's not the sexiest most

awesome thing in the world to do… but you do it anyway. It must get done.

You don't care what she thinks about it. That would be weird.

You just do it.

You're a big boy. The time of getting rewarded for going potty stopped decades ago

Mistake #3: Happy Wife, Happy Life

Wow, If I had a nickel for every time I've heard this stupid phrase.

In fact, I can think of one recent memory that involved myself, my kids, my wife and some random shoe store employee.

We needed shoes for my oldest boy (he was 10 at the time). We had an event coming up and he needed something nice but not too formal. He grew out of everything he had at home (like kids always seem to do)... so off to the mall we went!

We went to Macy's and decided to split up. My wife went to look at some dresses and my son and I went to the shoe department. We tried on a few pairs and found one that we both liked, but I wasn't sure about them and wanted my wife's input.

For one thing, I'm color-blind. Sometimes I don't see obvious color mismatches that make everyone else laugh uncontrollably. I honestly don't know if these shoes will go with the outfit that we already bought for our son.

Second, I can't trust my son to pick out something color-wise because, well, he was a 10-year-old boy at the time... and that means he had the fashion sense of a crazy man

42

with a bad cocaine habit.

The wife eventually wrapped up her dress shopping and met us at the shoes. We show her the one pair we both liked. She liked them, too… but, she didn't think it went too well with the outfit we bought for him. The shoelaces were a little too funky looking. Overall, the shoes were too sneaker-like, in her opinion. The style really limited what clothes he could wear with them.

Good point. We continued looking.

We walk into another shoe store and my wife grabs a pair off the shelf. "Here, these are much better." My son and I look at the shoes and blurt out at the same time, "They look JUST like the other pair!"

She points out that no, they are not JUST like the other pair. These have plain laces and not those speckled funny-looking laces the other pair had. These are overall more formal-looking. They look a little more sedate and will therefore have more options for matching clothes.

Ten seconds into our conversation, the guy running the shoe store loudly says in our direction, ***"Dude! Let me give you a hint! HAPPY WIFE, HAPPY LIFE!!"***

The message:

"Noooo! Don't have conflict with a woman! Let her win! Live another day, you poor man!"

How pathetic. After one very mild and normal exchange between my wife and I, this random shoe store worker was ready to throw in the towel for me. He was so unnerved by the site of a man disagreeing with a woman, that he had to come to my rescue. I can just picture him grabbing me by the hand and looking sullenly into my eyes, like a wise old man telling the hero of movie to not battle the evil Medusa. "Oh… you poor, poor man. Don't you realize what evil you are up against? Please… for your own sake, go back from where you came. You are not prepared for this battle."

What in the Sam Hell happened to men? Why are we all so conflict averse? Are we really that frightened of women? That's what we're saying after all, right… that we're legitimately afraid of them?

We're so afraid of women that many of us can't point out when we disagree with something. We let anger and resentment fester and turn into cancer and heart disease because … you don't want to make a scene? You don't want to make her mad?

Seriously?

"Yes, dear." – another common relationship trope. The resigned man. The droopy face. The slumped shoulders. The attitude that says, *"I don't care. Do whatever you like. Just stop being a bitch, ok? Please?"*

It's defeat. It's passivity. It's pathetic. It's a GIANT turnoff.

You think you're just being an adult and keeping the waters calm. You don't want to rock the boat unnecessarily. Your wife is far more emotional than you are, and you don't want to disrupt the current state of calm. One little thing can set her off. You've learned this over the years. When she does go off, she's a real handful. It's unattractive, annoying, brings about a great deal of anxiety and it makes you question the relationship. You'd prefer not to go there if you can help it.

You just want happiness and calm.

"Sigh... That's fine, honey."

What does she think of this reaction from you? Well, sure, she's happy at first. She gets her way. She's elated. Like a small child, she will say "Yaaaay!" and bounce around for a little while.

Over time, getting her way is just expected. The novelty is gone. Soon she won't even ask for your opinion on anything. She'll just do what she wants. She knows you wouldn't object anyway, so why delay the inevitable?

More importantly, one big thing happens:

She loses respect for you.

If she doesn't respect you, she's not fucking you.

When you try to avoid drama, what you're really trying to

avoid is your own anxiety. She makes you feel bad. Your emotional state should not be so fragile and pliable. You do your thing and let her emote. If her emotion crosses the line and she is disrespectful to you, you let her know immediately.

"You're being an asshole. Stop it. Now."

Believe it or not, she wants to be told NO every now and then. She sometimes really does want to be told to sit down, shut her mouth and stop acting like such a spoiled brat.

You are a dude. You are supposed to be a rock. You are supposed to be dependable. Sometimes that means welcoming confrontation and dealing with bullshit. Sometimes that bullshit comes from your own wife.

Doing the opposite elicits a feeling of disrespect, uncertainty, and disdain from her. That is NOT good for the female sex drive.

"So, wait… she doesn't like it when I submit and say 'Yes, dear' for the 500th time, but she'll also throw a huge fit if she doesn't get her way. Seriously? Why would she do this? I can't win!"
– Every guy who ever lived.

To try and help explain, a lot of men have concluded that this "bad" behavior from their wife is a type of test. You'll often hear them called "shit tests" or "fitness tests". Their purpose is to throw out something negative and then sit back and watch how you handle it. A sneaky way of saying,

"Show me what you got, big boy."

She's testing your boundaries. She wants to see what you're REALLY made of.

I've even heard some women flat out admit to consciously doing it.

Everyone, no matter what their gender, tests other people. We all do this consciously and subconsciously, and your wife is no different.

As your spouse, her tests are a way of seeing just how strong of a partner you really are. If you cave in to her demands, never stand up for yourself, refuse to make a decision, or freak out and pout after every little verbal tirade she has, what does that say about you?

"He can't deal with ME? Well then how the hell can he deal with the tough stuff in life? How can he protect me and the family? What kind of man is this?"

The result? Her innate programming sends signals to her body: *"This male is weak. Do not copulate. Genes not fit for mating."*

The result is no sexy time for you.

If she doesn't respect you, she's not fucking you.

What you are doing by saying "Yes, dear" for the hundredth time is being "agreeable".

Agreeableness is a personality trait that is most often seen in women. Women are more apt to be amicable, trusting, and compliant.

In other words, they are usually more submissive than men. Not always, of course, but usually.

When you just go with the flow and comply and submit to her every whim, you are being submissive. You are, in essence, acting like a woman.

She doesn't want a woman. She wants a man.

If she doesn't respect you, she's not fucking you.

Mistake #4: Pretend That No Other Females in the World Exist

If you're a man and you're healthy and everything is functioning as it should be, you have a relatively strong libido. You want to have sex. A lot. Obviously... or you wouldn't be reading this.

Biological fact: **You have evolved to procreate with a lot of different women.** You have about ten times the amount of testosterone that your wife has. Testosterone is the hormone that largely determines libido in human beings. Before you email me, yes, I realize human biology and psychology are not that simple and way more goes into sex drive than just one hormone... but, try taking a shot of testosterone every week for a month and get back to me on how it affects you (hint: you're going to be WAY hornier). I can remember reading the reaction of a woman who was prescribed testosterone therapy by her doctor: "This is crazy. I can't live like this. All I think about is sex."

As you read this, you are making sperm. Millions of them. Those little guys need to come out and they need to make babies to keep our species going. Mother nature made sure you do your part by imprinting you with basic programming that pushes you to do your job and to do it often.

This is the programming that makes you look at all those pretty young women at the mall. Repeatedly.

This is the programming that makes you keep looking at that MILF in the PTO meeting who just got the new boob implants.

This is the programming that makes pornography a billion-dollar industry.

Our sex drive is an essential part of us. It's THERE, and we live with it. It's natural. It's not going away. It's a big part of what makes us men.

Your wife knows this. She knows you masturbate to porn. She knows you fantasize. She caught you checking out that young girl the other day at the volleyball game. She probably said something about it. Depending on the health of your relationship, she may have even shamed you for it.

Men erroneously believe that once they are married, this drive and attraction to others must be hidden away. We think of ourselves as stupid horny animals. It seems that our community requires that we keep these urges at bay and channel that energy into our role as a family provider. To do otherwise means that we are encroaching on "asshole" territory, or worse… "unfit husband and dad".

So… how in the hell is your ever-present and much-maligned male sexuality supposed to fit into the preferred "provider" role?

It's frustrating.

Regardless of what society may tell us, these urges must come out, one way or another. If not, we lose our minds.

But wait a minute… what is this?? We have a woman in the house!? Our wife! Yes, of course! We love her! We even married her! Sweet! Let's get this show on the road.

You: "Honey! Let's have sex! It will be awesome!"
Her: "No."
You: "God dammit."

Now what? Well, if you're like most men out there, you know all the major porn video streaming websites by heart. You probably have a favorite category of video you like. A favorite "actress". Probably a few specific links you bookmarked. They seem to always get the job done in a hurry.

Then your wife sees your internet browser history. She doesn't like it. You're supposed to not like those things anymore, remember? Did you forget your role in life? What kind of man and father are you? Why are you watching this stuff? Fucking cut it out already, you sicko pervert.

You have been shamed.

The sex life has tanked. Porn is shameful. What the hell can you do!?

You know what to do! You'll take things up a notch. You feel that she probably doubts your attraction to her and questions your faithfulness. You'll show her that she's dead wrong. In fact, you don't NEED all that outside stimuli anymore. You'll show her how devoted you are to her and only her!

You'll show her your softer, more romantic side! She likes that!

You'll show her that no other woman on the planet exists but HER!

Then she will realize what a romantic you really are, she'll remember why she fell in love with you, and your sex life will be reignited.

Yeah... no.

Just like with your fear of confrontation (happy wife, happy life), you are pretending. You are withholding your true feelings, your true NATURE, with the underhanded purpose of getting affection from your wife.

She knows what you're really all about. She's been aware of the true sexual nature of men since she went into puberty and suddenly sprouted boobs. She knows you have urges. You've probably reminded her of your needs on numerous occasions.

By tempering these urges and professing that SHE ALONE holds the key to your manly human nature (with or without actual sex from her), you are putting her right up on a pedestal.

She has no option but to look down on you.

If she doesn't respect you, she's not fucking you.

Here's a very common "shit test" scenario:

You and your wife are watching TV. It's one of those "Bachelor" reality shows where the hunky lover guy gets to go on dates and pick from a harem of attractive women. One will eventually be chosen, and the lucky girl gets to be his girlfriend or even fiancée.

It's woman porn, basically.

Wife: "Which girl do you think looks the best?"

Husband: "Oh, I dunno."

Wife: "No, tell me. Which one would you pick if you were him? Be honest."

Husband: *sweating profusely* "Ummm… well… the blond one looks a lot like you. You have better legs, though."

Wife: "Ha! You're so full of shit. She's like TWENTY years old and is flawless. She's an Olympic track athlete! I've never had legs like that. I haven't been to the gym in like 15 years."

Husband: "Oh, well, I think you're beautiful the way you are."

Wife: "The way I am? What the hell is that supposed to mean? How AM I, exactly?"

Husband: "Sigh…"

Test FAILED.

As you can see in this scenario, even the well-intentioned lie backfires. She sniffed out his bullshit right away. She knows he finds those women attractive and she knows she's no spring chicken anymore. Instead of being honest, the man starts mumbling and spazzing out like some nerdy teenager getting caught jerking off in the bathroom.

Admitting your attraction to others is not shameful. You haven't been "caught" doing something bad. Take pride in your sexuality.

Here's how that conversation would go between my wife and I:

Wife: "Which girl do you think looks the best?"

Me: "Hmmmm… I like the brunette. There's something sexy about her. She has a nice body but looks a little rough around the edges. I bet she's kinky, though. The red head is a little chubby but pretty. She has that girl next door look. Hmmmm… tough decision. Probably the brunette."

Wife: "Yeah, but the brunette is just a few years away from

looking really rough. Kinda crazy, too. Not good wife material. I like the blond."

Me: "Oh, I wasn't thinking wife material. I'm thinking of just a few hours of fun. She would get annoying really fast. She's nuttier than squirrel poop."

Wife: "Haha! Yep."

See the difference? It's light-hearted, honest, and playful. It's fun but sexy talk.

Ok, but what if a husband was being honest and it backfired on him?

Wife: "You know what… You're an asshole. If you had asked me about a bunch of guys I would say none of them looked good. I don't care about other men. Apparently, you care about other women a whole lot."

Husband: "HAHAHA. Well, you asked!"

Wife: "Whatever."

Wife is pissed. Wife pouts.

The strong, honest and attractive husband doesn't care. He thinks it's hilarious. Why should he take this seriously? He answered her damn question. If she was fishing for comfort and lies instead of truth, she can go talk to her girlfriends. Her man is a rock and is there to be honest. She can count on him to be truthful, even when it hurts. Especially about a silly thing like which girl is the prettiest on a TV reality show.

The moment will blow over. It's no big deal.

"Which girl do you think looks the best?" = "Are you willing to be honest with me and with yourself even if it means hurting my feelings? Can you handle the possible nagging and anger that will result, or will you fold like a little baby?"

Remember: If a man can't be true to himself, he can't be true to others. He's untrustworthy. He's a slimy wuss. You always want to err on the side of integrity and honesty. Always.

A wife knows that her man is sexual. She knows he's attracted to other women. A LOT of other women. He wants to have sex with them. Duh. He's a man. He doesn't go out and fornicate with a bunch of women because he is married and devoted to his wife. He's making a sacrifice. She knows it. You know it. Stop changing reality to accommodate her feelings. Stop tip-toeing around her. Stop walking on eggshells. It's ok if she's pissed off. It's not the end of the world.

Want to gauge just how sexually attracted your wife is to you? Have somebody ask her:

"How quickly do you think your husband could get another woman and have sex with her?"

Does she laugh? That means you're not a sexual being in her eyes. You're a provider that she lost respect for and no longer sees as a sexual being. You have a lot of work ahead of you.

Does she get worried or angry at the idea? She knows you're attractive and a good catch. Your resources and partnership could easily go bye-bye.

Does she get turned on? Well then, what the hell are you doing reading this book? She's a horn dog and is crazy about you!

The man who other women find attractive is attractive to his wife. The man who could go out and get sex next week is a guy who is frequently banging his wife.

"He could have a lot of other pretty women, but he chose me."

This is rare in a husband these days. Rare is good. That's your goal. A big part of reaching that goal is being a strong man of integrity.

Mistake #5: Talk Talk Talk Talk

Alright, you've tried romantic gifts of appreciation, you've upped your chore game, you're much more agreeable and you've reassured her that there is no other woman that even comes remotely close to turning you on like she does.

Didn't work, did it? Your sex life seems to be stuck on terrible. No passion. No oomph. At best, your wife is giving you pity sex to shut you up.

Now what do you do? Call it quits? Leave her? Find somebody new?

Well, again… you're a dude. You're not done tinkering around under the hood of the car. You're determined to figure out why this engine is misfiring so badly.

You ask around for advice. Close friends. The internet. Maybe a therapist.

One thing is repeated again and again by everyone:

COMMUNICATION.

When you feel a certain way, you should just tell her, right? Makes sense. That's what adults do. We get issues out in the open and talk about them until they are resolved. Give and take. Compromise. This is part of any good partnership.

You want sex. It's important to you. She obviously doesn't

feel the same way. Maybe this is the natural state for a wife/mom to be in, and you just need to remind her that couples are supposed to have sex. Maybe she just legitimately forgets about the importance of physical intimacy.

Maybe she doesn't understand just HOW important this is to you. Maybe if you sit her down and nicely explain how hurt you are by this lack of intimacy, she will suddenly comply and start her sexual engine up again for you.

Ultimately, physical intimacy is a choice, right?

So, if you're like most men, you eventually cave in to your frustration and tell her how you feel. She listens. She gets a little emotional as you pour your guts out to her. She seems genuinely surprised that you were so hurt by this. She says you have sex at least once every couple of weeks…isn't that enough? You explain to her that you started keeping track of sex and it's been two months since your last session. Before that, there was a three-month break. She seems puzzled by this. "Are you sure it's been that long?"

Obviously, this sexual drought doesn't have the same negative impact on her.

You feel a glimmer of hope, though. You can see that the severity of this situation is starting to sink in a bit. You are getting somewhere. You press on.

You explain that you are bothered by her apparent lack of desire for you. Nothing you do ever turns her on. You're always turned on by HER, but she can't seem to be able to muster up the energy to reciprocate. ***"Is it that you just don't love me anymore?"***

She starts crying and explaining.

She's under stress, she says. The house. The kids. Work. It's all just too much to bear at times. All of these things prevent her from getting into the headspace necessary for sexual arousal. She never even thinks about sex. It's not you, it's her. "Just be patient and understanding with me. Ok?"

You hold her. You tell her you're sorry. You'll help more around the house. You'll get the kids three days a week after school instead of two. You'll be there more for her, emotionally. You've not been the best partner. You can do better.

She appreciates your help and thanks you for being such a great husband and friend.

You kiss. You hug a while. More crying. She gets up to make dinner. You run off to play with the kids.

Later that night, you go to bed and see her already asleep under the covers. You give her a gentle kiss and go to the basement with your laptop and jerk off to porn. Again.

Still, if you're being honest, you DO feel a lot better about your situation. Communication is important, after all. It feels good to get all that off your chest. You finally feel like you may be moving the relationship in the right direction.

Another month will go by. No sex. You will decide to have the talk again.

Subsequent conversations with your wife won't be so sweet. She'll become more frustrated with you. The emotional façade goes away and is replaced with anger and annoyance.

At times, she seems almost repulsed by your touch. Even the most innocent of back rubs and kisses make her stiffen up.

It feels like you are roommates, or worse… siblings.

More talking. More emotional vomiting. More anger. The cycle continues.

Hammer this into your head: **The talk doesn't work.**

The talk just reaffirms what she already knows deep down: **You are not the kind of guy she wants to fuck.**

What you are doing is looking for her help. You're asking her to fix the problem. You are putting yourself in a subservient role. You are like a child looking up to mom to fix his booboo.

This is a gigantic female libido killer.

Each talk just drives one thing into her brain: ***"Oh God. I married a guy who just doesn't GET IT and he probably*** *never will."*

When you pour your guts out to your wife, you're trying to appeal to her rational side.

"Don't you remember how much we love each other? Remember all our good times? Remember all those loving and romantic feelings we have for each other? Intimacy is a choice. I love you and choose to want you sexually ALL the time. I don't understand why you refuse to make the same decision."

Instead of appealing to her rational mind, you are setting off an instinctual response that pushes the libido in the wrong direction. Rationality doesn't enter into the world of eroticism and animalistic desire that you want and need so badly. Having "the talk" with your wife is like walking into the middle of a funeral and performing a strip tease.

If the talk was truly an open and honest conversation, it would go something like this:

You: *"Why don't we have sex more?"*

Her: *"Because you don't turn me on."*

You: *"Okay, what do I need to do to turn you on more?"*

Her: *"If I have to tell you what to do, then it turns me off even more. You should just know what to do. I want a guy who just KNOWS."*

You: *"Well then there's no hope for me, right?"*

Her: *"Probably not. Up to you."*

You: *"So, is that it? We should just divorce?"*

Her: *"Maybe, but that would be ugly and cost us a lot of money and cause the kids irreparable long-term harm. How about instead we just keep this up for a while until one of us has an affair?"*

You: *"Alright, cool. I'll be in the basement."*

Her: *"Okay. Enjoy jerking off. Loser."*

Everything else said in the talk is just bullshit. The talk is just two people tap-dancing around the bigger picture.

Everyone is ignoring the elephant in the room: She just isn't turned on.

The TALK is one of the worst things you can do to try and reignite sexual desire.

I understand you have a lot of things on your mind and feel sad and you want to let your partner know. The problem is that she doesn't like being emotionally dumped on by her man. She certainly doesn't want to be reminded of how she no longer has sexual desire for you.

For her, the world already feels like it's spinning out of control at times. She wasn't lying about all the pressure she's under. Sometimes it is just too much. You're just adding to the stress of life instead of being the escape she wants and needs so badly.

She doesn't want YOUR problems on top of the giant pile of her OWN problems. Especially when the underlying cause of your problems can be summed up as, *"You know... you're kind of a shitty wife."*

Yes, she complains about everything to you ALL THE FUCKING TIME. Yes, you should be able to do the same when it comes to your lack of sex. No, you cannot. Yes, it's a double-standard. Yes, it's sexist. Sorry, that's real life. Why do you think men for centuries have bottled up their insecurities and emotions and only have deep talks with select guy friends?

Because nobody else, especially your wife, will give a shit about you not getting the sex you feel you so richly deserve.

"But, that's not what she said."

Your wife may ask you to please open up to her and trust her with your feelings. She may say she doesn't feel close as a couple unless you let her know what's going on with you and why you're so down lately.

Don't do it.

First of all, she absolutely knows what is going on in your head. You've been begging her for sex in one way or another for quite some time. Again, she knows that men are usually way more horny than women. It's not some well-kept secret. To her, everything you do at home seems to revolve around trying to get in her pants.

So then, why would she ask you to open up if she doesn't want to hear it?

Because this is another one of those TESTS.

Almost every married man has experienced something similar to this scenario:

Her: *"Please tell me what is wrong. I'm your wife. You need to share these things with me. I love you. I'm here for you."*

Him: *"OK…well.."* [insert massive amounts of emotional vomiting here]

Her: *"Well… I'm going to need some time alone to process this. Just… no… don't touch me right now. Just… leave me alone for a while."*

Your wife is not wired to listen to her man endlessly emote.

To quote author and psychotherapist Esther Perel:

"Men are afraid of women's tensions, but women are afraid of men's meltdowns—that they will regress, suddenly going

from man to boy to baby. Women believe that men are more fragile on some fundamental level, and they think that if they let loose, they'll fall apart. Many women don't trust in the emotional resilience of men. They think they are superior in this realm.

Many women are also afraid that if they soften their partner, then they won't be able lean on him. They fundamentally still want him to be strong, because that allows them to fall apart: I need to know that you can hold me and that you're strong. If you're not strong, I can't let go. This is true in sex and this is true emotionally. If/when for some reason he softens, there is a part of her that feels angry. Instead of becoming compassionate, she becomes angry."

Your wife is especially not wired to listen to her husband complain about what she already knows deep down inside: He doesn't turn her on.

You might as well sit her down, start crying and repeatedly yell in her face, **"I'M NOT ATTRACTIVE! I'M NOT ATTRACTIVE! I'M NOT ATTRACTIVE!"**

She would LOVE to come home every day to a rock of a man who is strong no matter what is going on in the world. She wants a guy she can collapse into. Somebody to make her feel safe and loved.

Instead, she has this whiny little husband that is repeatedly asking her for sex and yapping about his nonsense, like a

Chihuahua begging for scraps from the dinner table.

Not good. Not manly. Not attractive. Very needy.

When you talk to your woman about her lack of libido, you might as well be talking to the sky about the lack of rain. You'll get the same result.

Yes, after much whining, your wife may eventually throw you a bone just to shut you up. She'll finally cave in and have the dreaded "pity sex" with you. *"Fine... let's do this. But hurry up, my show is coming on in 10 minutes."*

But, if we're being honest, we don't like it. Not at all. We really don't want a lifeless mannequin lying in bed with her legs open saying, "Fuck me. Please. You stallion. Take me. Oh god. Yes." as she blankly stares off into space, like some sarcastic monotone robot.

We want passion.
We want to be desired.
We want a woman who can't help herself.
We want to feel like a man again.

TALKING and rationalizing with your wife will never bring this about.

You're thinking like a dude. "I want sex every day. I have a penis. You have a vagina. I'm turned on just thinking about it. Let's do this."

Remember, you are engineered to do this. You get erect if the wind blows just right. In case you couldn't tell, your wife is not built the same.

From a strictly biological standpoint, libido is largely governed by testosterone. You have roughly TEN TIMES the amount of testosterone that she does. This is what gives you the deeper voice, body hair, stronger bones, muscles and the desire to bang all those giggling 18-year old girls you saw at the movies last weekend.

To get your wife's engine going requires a delicate recipe akin to a soufflé. One wrong move and the whole thing collapses.

You've been making wrong moves for years now. One little chat is not going to resolve this. Hundreds of chats won't result in carnal desire.

We're talking about emotion. Nature. Human nature. Our innate programming. You can't beat that with reason and logic.

Stop trying. Stop talking.

The programming doesn't give a shit.

CHAPTER 3
"Nice Guys" Finish Last

"If you're ever yelling at a woman, all you should be saying is, 'Why can't you be my mommy? Why are you NOT my mommy?'"

Marc Maron

The Five Mistakes All Have One Thing in Common

Their methods and expected outcomes are not grounded in reality. They are all grounded in the world of what SHOULD be. They're all from the typical "Nice Guy" book of rules.

X does not seem to result in Y… but, dammit, it should!

This concept of "should" is getting you nowhere in life.

You're stomping your feet like a child and screaming **"IT'S NOT FAIR! I'M A REALLY GREAT GUY!! WHERE'S MY SEX?!"** How's that working out for you?

You are attempting to apply your logic, reason, and a sense of right and wrong to a world where the most basic and instinctual behavior reigns supreme.

You can't out-nice her lack of sexual desire.

The world of sexual desire is governed by instinct. It's controlled by thousands and thousands of years of programming that is deeply embedded into our DNA.

Sometimes, the programming is predictable.

"If young pretty woman with nice skin and a sexy shape looks at me, smiles and plays with her hair - Then activate erection sequence for quick copulation."

71

Sometimes, the programming is confusing.

"If skinny, androgynous heroin-addicted rock star looks at me -> Then pump blood to vulva to increase chances of successful intercourse and fertilization."

But, there's absolutely nothing in that programming that says:

"If sweet, well-intentioned male that promised to love me unconditionally forever asks me for sex -> Then activate immediate fornication sequence."

This programming is not nice. It is not politically correct. It does not care about you and your feelings. It doesn't take into consideration the last 100 years of progressive societal change. In evolutionary terms, that's a fraction of a blink of an eye.

The programming certainly doesn't care about your past 10 years of being a great dad and loving partner. The programming laughs at your Nice Guy behavior.

Yes, the programming is a major asshole.

And yet, we all think we can outsmart this programming, don't we? I certainly don't blame you for trying. We seem to control everything else around us, so why not human sexuality? Surely, we can rise above the shallowness of the caveman programming and become deeper, more thoughtful human beings and set aside all this shallow bullshit, right?

Unfortunately, no. We keep trying to rewrite the programming… and we keep failing. We may have temporary success (awful pity sex), but the end result is the same: The wife is just even more turned off than before.

Been there, done that, along with millions of other men.

The five mistakes are rooted in the belief that the sexual machine we have in us is inherently moral. We think we live day-to-day in a world that that we can manipulate via our free will. We extend that mindset to matters where it's laughably wrong.

We think our wife has a choice of whether or not to be sexually aroused.

She doesn't.

Yes, she can physically walk to the bedroom, take off her clothes, open her legs and say "Go ahead. Get it over with." What she can't do it flip on the switch that turns on TRUE sexual desire.

Going through the motions does not mean she is aroused. It just means she's trying to shut you up and get it over with so she can move on to more important things.

You don't want that. None of us want that.

It's time to throw in the towel and listen to the primal machine for once. It's not going anywhere.

It's been there for thousands of generations.

You Can't "Nice" Your Way Into Her Pants

To illustrate: I don't care what kind of flirtatious skills or awesome personality she may have, I cannot get aroused by a 900-pound woman with a beard. She can tell me what a dirty slut she is, and how she won the "Best blowjobs in Texas" award 10 years in a row … but she can't overcome my innate programming that screams, "RUN FOR YOUR LIFE!!".

Same rule applies to your situation.

"Dude… are you calling me a 900-pound bearded woman?"

Yes. Yes, I am.

I don't care how many bags of trash you take out, how many purses you buy her, what kind of fancy SUV you lease for her, how many long and deep conversations about your awful sex life you may have… These things just can't get her sexual engine going.

In fact, they may put you further down in the shitty hole you are trying to escape from. Why? Because you just don't get it. Her programming wants somebody who GETS it. Her programming is looking for a match to its primal needs. The more you keep committing the same mistakes, the more you just reinforce the negative instinctual response she has lingering deep in her programming.

No wonder you're in a dead bedroom.

Let's be honest… Your wife loves you. She appreciates all you do for her and the kids. She values your friendship and partnership over the years. She may indeed consider you the love of her life. She may plan to live with you until the day she dies.

None of that can overcome the hindbrain sending her repeated signals that say **"ABORT SEXUAL RESPONSE. THIS MALE IS NOT FIT FOR REPRODUCTION."** Those signals may not be strong enough for her to divorce you, but those signals are what keep her comfy sweatpants on night after night.

Nothing can reverse that programming… except somebody that truly does turn her on.

You simply want her to look at you, bite her lip, take her clothes off, and drag you into the bedroom?

That is a primal reaction. This requires primal action on your part.

You can't drag desire out of her with kindness and understanding.

It sucks… but it's true.

Nice guys do, in fact, finish last.

Stop Putting the Poor Woman on a Pedestal

Look, I get it. You're a good man. You have a good heart. You love your wife and you just want that passion back again. You're having a hard time balancing your basic horny male programming with your rational brain telling you that you love your wife and she's your best friend, partner, mom to your kids, etc.

This doesn't change the fact that she's every bit as flawed as you are. You have worshiped this poor woman for far too long.

Your wife farts. She takes dumps. She gets pimples. She has wrinkles. She has cellulite. She smells bad if she doesn't shower. She's also completely devoid of superpowers. In fact, she is probably physically weaker than you are.

She's a human being.

I know... you've been told to always be a gentleman. Treat her like a queen. "Happy wife, happy life". She's the fairer sex, after all. A delicate flower that requires great care. You need to keep your stew of toxic masculinity on a low simmer or else you'll risk being an abusive asshole and scare her away.

This "soft" theme permeates your actions as well as your results.

Your gifts, your chore play, your lying, your tip-toeing, your constant talking and seeking reassurance… They all have the theme of *"Please, your highness, am I now worthy of your affection?"*

It's all a variation on one theme: **Neediness.**

Every time you try one of the five mistakes, you are striking the proverbial chisel. Piece by piece, you are building a marble effigy in your wife's image. The placard on the front reads, *"My wife. She's now a giant bitch that never wants sex with me. I still worship her, though. I need her. Without her, I am lost."*

Contrary to popular belief, she doesn't want to be the ruler of your world. She doesn't want you to worship her. She doesn't want you to NEED her. She wants YOU to be the marble statue, not her. She wants to be able to point across the crowded room and say to her friends, *"That's MY MAN right there!"*

How can she look up to you and respect you if she's looking down on you?

If she doesn't respect you, she's not fucking you.

"My wife told me that she loves my good-natured sweet side. She told me she wants to see more of that. She likes it when I cater to her. She hates it when I act any other way. She says that turns her off and ruins any chance we have

for future sex."

Listen to her… smile… and observe.

What she DOES is far more important than what she SAYS.

Or, in your case, what she's NOT doing (having sex with you) is more important than what she says. You're listening to a woman who is not attracted to you tell you that the key to her attraction is to "keeping being you".

That makes zero sense.

Do you want me to share the countless stories from men who started snooping on their cold sexless wives and found dirty diaries and photos of them doing crazy, now forbidden sexual acts with ex-boyfriends. She was able to get to that elusive erotic headspace with "losers" from her past, but she just can't bring herself to do the same with her loving and devoted husband of twenty years. *"I was a different girl back then. I've changed!"*

Do you want to hear about the guy who could never get his wife to do oral sex with him because she said that it was "gross" and "that sort of thing is for porn", only to find a video of her having a threesome last week with a guy and another woman from her Crossfit class?

How about the countless sexually-frustrated men who stare angrily at their wives' well-worn vibrators and growing stack of filthy romance novels.

Your wife has sexual/intimacy needs, too. She's a human being. Right now, those needs are either dormant and waiting to come out for the right guy, or they are already out and she is screwing around behind your back.

"But, she said..."

She will SAY whatever she feels you want to hear. Your actions over the years have probably told her that you are a pretty sensitive guy. She doesn't want to see a pouty whining man sulking around the house... so she keeps her true feelings to herself. You can think of this as her version of "happy wife happy life." A whiny and beaten man makes her anxious and sometimes very angry. She'd prefer to not go to that emotional space, if possible. Saying, "It's not you, it's me" or "Just be you" keeps you at bay.

If you are wealthy Mr. Provider Extraordinaire, or best dad in the universe, then she REALLY doesn't want to rock the relationship boat. She has a good thing going. "It's not you, it's me" buys her more time. Maybe she'll throw you some pity sex to keep you quiet for a while. She must keep the Provider's resource machine humming along.

On the other hand, she truly may NOT know why she has no desire for you anymore. All she knows is that the switch got turned off some time ago and nothing seems to be able to turn it back on. Sex just isn't on her mind anymore. "Maybe I'm just asexual" she says, or worse, "Maybe I'm a broken person".

A surprisingly large number of women are completely clueless about what gets their sexual engine going. Ironically, they too feel like they SHOULD be aroused and ready to have sex with their husband… but man, they just can't muster the energy and bring about the mindset necessary to get to that level of intimacy and eroticism with their loving spouse. Faking it and pity sex kills them inside just as much as it does for the husband.

Many women will openly talk about sex with their friends. They will report back to the husband (after enduring one of his many talks): *"A lot of women are like me. We just don't want sex that much after we have kids. It's natural. There's nothing wrong with that."* Yes, it is perfectly natural and predictable behavior. That is until somebody else comes along and gets their sexual engine going again. That sexual reawakening is just as natural and just as predictable.

My experience shows that when these "low libido" women DO wake up from their sexual slumber…oh boy. Watch out. "Sexual deviance" doesn't begin to cover it. "Slut" is not a strong enough word.

That's when men who discover an affair find themselves saying, *"This isn't my wife. She's acting crazy."*

No, it's your wife. It's always been your wife. She's not "crazy". She's in love. She's turned on. People in love sometimes do wacky, irrational stuff. They make some major life mistakes. They move across country. They quit their jobs. They act foolish and irresponsible. They are like crazy and rebellious teenagers. They also have lots of sex.

You want to generate this type of "crazy" response in your wife. **She wants that, too.**

Big Picture Question: Do You, Mr. Nice Guy, REALLY Want Sex From Your Wife?

Two big questions you need to ask yourself:

1. Do you REALLY want your wife?

2. Are you REALLY willing to make the changes needed to improve your sex life?

Let's first break down question number one. Here's a common scenario I hear from men that I chat with during one-on-one sessions (you can book your own session with me at dadstartingover.com):

Reader: *"Man my wife is just awful. She does all of these horrible things on a regular basis. Let me tell you about these twelve terrible awful things she did just yesterday."*

Me: *"Okay, yeah… that's all pretty awful. So, what is your goal here with this relationship?"*

Reader: *"Well, I read The Dead Bedroom Fix, so obviously I want more sex from my wife."*

Let's stop and think about this. The man just told me, in grueling detail, about just what an awful human being his wife is. His next thought: "So… where's my sex?"

The kicker in these scenarios is that the wife KNOWS she is not a good wife. She KNOWS she is treating her husband poorly. She KNOWS that she has been building a case for winning the "worst wife ever" prize year after year. And yet... here comes Mr. Erection again. "So... wanna have sex?"

What does that mean to the wife? *"He doesn't actually want ME, he just wants sexual gratification."* Basically, you want to use your wife as a big angry masturbation device. In her mind, there's no attempt at real connection. There's no real effort to become somebody that she actually wants. There's no longer any attempt at playing the mating game in any way... beyond just pressuring her so that you can use her as a warm hole.

Does your wife fit into this scenario? Do you, in fact, just want to use her to fulfill your needs... rather than you wanting her because of your genuine lust and desire for HER as a person? When she walks across the room, do you find your eyes following her and saying to yourself, "God, she is so gorgeous"? When she does something for you and the family, do you look at her and say, "She is one amazing wife. I just love her to death"? Do you have genuine love, admiration, appreciation, and lust for your wife?

It surprises me how many men hesitate at this line of questioning. What should be a knee jerk response of ,"Yes, of course! I'm crazy about her!" is instead one of quiet realization. *"Wow... I really don't like my wife."*

84

If this is your case, you have a lot of work to do. You have a lot of introspection and deep thinking to do about you, your relationship, and your future as either her husband or as a newly single man.

Now, on to question number two: **Are you REALLY willing to make the changes needed to improve your sex life?"**

Let's assume that you do still have genuine love, admiration, appreciation, and lust for your wife. Don't think for a minute that things will be much easier for you. The question I have posed may seem silly (after all, you bought this book, right?), but we're talking about altering your reality here. We're talking about doing stuff that is mostly likely WAY outside of your comfort zone. I can't stress enough how, for many of you, this will be a complete 180 from how you have done things up to this point in your marriage.

Some guys get into this process and later say, "Alright… you know what? Nope. Not happening. I'm going back to the old me." Years later they are still where they were before, or worse.

It's not going to be easy. Not at all.

You gotta have balls to make real change. Courage. The willingness to fail again and again. You must set aside your "fragile male ego". You can't tip toe your way out of this mess.

Think of a skill that you have practiced for years. Something you consider yourself to be pretty good at. For me, it would be photography and videography. I've been taking photos for over 20 years now. I would consider myself to be up-to-date on all the latest technology. I'm well versed on the technical side of things … ISO, depth of field, white balance, shutter speed, the rule of thirds, etc.

I have a good eye for aesthetics and what makes a "good" photo.

Still, somebody out there knows A HELL OF A LOT more than me. I watch a Philip Bloom video and say, "Dammit… I suck." It's a blow to the ego.

As far as my little world of clients and friends are concerned, I get the job done. I'm pretty damn good. "Wow… you did that?!"

As far as the rest of the world is concerned, I'm average. I have a lot to learn still.

That's not a bad thing. Learning is good. Sometimes it means setting aside my preconceived notions of how to do something. I just need to shut up, listen and learn.

Mentors are amazing. They are worth their weight in gold. They can save you from committing tons of mistakes and they allow you to get results you wouldn't otherwise get… and get them much faster.

So, with the mentor philosophy in mind, is there anybody

else who would be a great "Get sex from women" mentor? No? Can't think of a single person? Are you sure about that?

Think back on your life from puberty, up until today. Remember your teen years. Who got all of the girls? Who was Mr. Popular? Which kid in school got laid first? How about in college? Who was just swimming in coeds and had to beat them off with a stick? Who would always sneak girls over to their dorm room? Who has the happy sexy MILF of a wife that all the other dads drool over?

Got the image of the guy in mind? What do all these guys have in common? What do they DO? To get your wife's engine going again, you will need to emulate some basic behaviors that you have, ironically, observed your whole life. That's right, you were given up-close lessons on how to score sex for YEARS, but you ignored them, or at the very least downplayed their importance.

Those same lessons apply now to your marriage.

The steps you must take to generate desire are steps that you have continuously dismissed as shallow, stupid, manipulative, and archaic. You have convinced yourself that you are above the silly stuff.

"I don't play games."

"Ha! I don't have to do that stuff... I'm married."

Oh yeah? No games? You're above that bullshit? Ok, cool.

How's that working out for you?

Exactly.

Set aside your prejudices. Ignore your advanced college degree. Forget what mom told you.

Pretend you don't have a cultured, more enlightened, and morally superior outlook on life, love and marriage… and just listen. You don't have to listen to me. You can follow the endless examples you see around you every single day.

I'll be honest…I'm a real softy. I'm a sensitive dude. I'm your quintessential "sweet" guy. I love babies, cute animals, playing with my kids, art, photography, music, romance… and I always have. That's me. I'm not talking about changing who you are. I'm talking about stepping out of your comfort zone and recognizing that sometimes you must do things completely different to get the result you want.

Sometimes that means setting aside what you think is "good" and "kind" (it's very often not).
We're going back to high school level stuff here. We're going over the stuff that dad or your older brother should've taught you but didn't. Maybe they did try, but their advice was drowned out by well-intentioned girls and friends telling you to "just be yourself."

Sound like I'm talking about dating or how to pick up girls? Yeah… we are, in a sense. What, you thought all that ended when you got married? You thought you would "outgrow" all that silly BS?

Not even close, cowboy.

You need that silly BS now more than ever.

It's okay, we've all been there. Some of us learn the lesson the hard way. Some of us never get that chance and we die after having decades of a mediocre and unfulfilling sex life and marriage. Some of us learn that our wife was a super sexual person… but only with other men. Some of us learn that our wife fell out of love with us years ago and only hung around for the paycheck.

NOT you, though. You're going to say, "To hell with all that." You're going to turn this around.

CHAPTER 4
Be Her Lover

"A successful marriage requires falling in love many times, always with the same person.'"

Mignon McLaughlin

Years ago, shortly after my divorce, I was at my oldest boy's wrestling practice chatting with another dad. We were roughly the same age. He said he noticed me lifting weights the other day at the gym we both attended. He told me he was just doing cardio at the time to lose weight, but he was impressed with my weightlifting.

Then he does what all out-of-shape older guys do: He started bragging about how he USED to be Awesome Mr. Weightlifter Guy back in the day.

Him: *"I could bench 315 for 10 reps when I was in college."*

Wow. Never heard that one before.

I indulge him a little. I tell him that he was stronger than I've ever been. I tell him that now I skip the bench press and use dumbbells instead because of my shoulder pain, how I need to stretch way more, takes me longer to recuperate…

He cuts me off. He doesn't want to hear it.

Him: **"Yeah, well… I don't have to do any of that shit anymore. I'm married."**

See, he knew I was divorced and dating at the time. My wife leaving me was a big event in our small circle of wrestling parents.

Here's the subtext of what he was really saying:

"You have to do all that building and maintaining your body because you are looking for a new woman. I already have one. No need to keep up the charade."

There's an understood dynamic at play in the post-divorce/single dating world. We instinctively recognize our need to lower our "Provider" traits and amplify our "Lover" traits. We hit the gym, dress nicer, get more frequent haircuts, get a sportier car, etc. All of this gives the appearance of being "fun" and "good looking". We know that if we want the girl of our dreams, we must look and play the part of the "Lover". After all, we're in hunting mode. We instinctively know the best way to attract our prey.

You don't approach a pretty little thing at the bar and say, "I'm really good at ironing and folding laundry."

Later, when we finally land a woman and marry her, the universal understanding is that you must now flip the scales in favor of Provider mode. You can let the stupid Lover stuff go… It's no longer needed. We, as men, must then focus on being a Provider above all else. We must now understand our new role in life and devote ourselves completely to it.

It's our own form of the classic "bait and switch".

This is the wrong thing to do on so many levels.

You want to be your wife's Lover. Always. If you're not, then somebody or something else will give her that emotional and physical high that she needs.

Saying "I do" shouldn't change your mating habits. In fact, ironically, it means that you must ramp up your Lover qualities even more. Why? Because now that she has a committed husband, your wife will also start to naturally get more comfortable. In the world of the woman's libido, comfort does not correspond to sexual desire. I repeat:

COMFORT DOES NOT EQUAL SEXUAL DESIRE.

But, wait… comfort is what you want to provide, right? You want to help put a roof over her head. Food on the table. Be there for her when things go wrong. Help her when she is sick, right?

Yes, of course. Keep doing those things. They're wonderful things. That's part of being an awesome human. This is the essence of being a good life partner.

But realize that these things don't result in a horny wife. You can't just put all your eggs in the Provider basket and hope for porn star level of activity in the bedroom.

A romantic relationship that is built solely on Provider points is not sustainable.

The Marriage Landscape Has Drastically Changed

Guys, some of you are playing by a very old and outdated book of marriage rules. I'm sorry to have to break this to you, but the 1950's are over. Full-time housewives are a very rare thing. In fact, women are now more educated than ever. Women make up the majority of our university graduates. They are career focused. They excel at their jobs and reach high levels of performance and rank within their companies. Suzy Homemaker is not completely dead, but she's on life support.

Does this new role in life make women happier and more fulfilled human beings? No, of course not. They are as unhappy as ever (welcome to the pointless rat race, ladies). What it does do is give them more options in life. Having more freedom reinforces the concept of, *"I really don't have to live like this if I don't want to."*

We know ladies are fickle by nature. One day she loves something... the next day she hates it with a burning passion and has a completely rational (and lengthy) explanation as to why she has a sudden change of heart.

Now, apply this same fickle mindset to marriage.

Women initiate 70% of divorce. If they're not happy... they're leaving and taking their BMW with them.

The days of the man coming home from a long day at work, taking his hat off and expecting a stiff drink and a hot meal waiting for him are long gone. There's no innate reward for being the breadwinner with the penis. He must find other ways to earn the title of "good husband". The paycheck and pointless job title just don't cut it anymore. She already has or can have those things, too. In fact, for many of you, your wife makes more money than you… or has the capacity to do so. She's one promotion away from leaving you in the dust.

What if you do happen to make more money than her? Unfortunately, as many of my readers have learned, there are these little things called "divorce", "alimony", and "child support" that can very quickly take care of that. Millions of men have discovered this awesome trifecta of soul-crushing state-mandated resource allocation.

The wife doesn't have to endure a boring and unfulfilling marriage anymore. All the barriers between her and a more fulfilling life have been eliminated. She's a free woman.

Want to be in a happy and sexual relationship with one woman for the rest of your life? You got your work cut out for you, amigo.

Women Are Having Affairs Now More Than Ever

Many men that visit my site and reach out to me have experienced the pain of discovering their wife's affair. A big percentage of those affairs were precipitated by some type of life-altering event that served as the relationship tipping point. Sometimes it was stressful and terrible (like death or illness), but many times it was something simple like the wife landing a big promotion at work.

Something simple like a little extra money in her paycheck was the straw that broke the marriage camel's back.

It's really very simple: At some point in the relationship, she naturally lost sexual interest in her husband (comfort and boredom set in), but she stayed with him for the familiarity, security, and resources. Then, through her own hard work, she achieved the ability to make her own money. She then has an epiphany. There is no longer a "need" for her husband.

"He's not a fun…He doesn't turn me on… I don't really like him all that much anymore… I make more money than he does… So, what am I doing with him again?"

That's when she lets her guard down and allows her buttons to be so easily pushed. Her programming has been activated. "Must find new mate". Ironically, she usually runs off and has an affair with a man who, by pretty much everyone's standards, is a complete and total loser.

Everyone: *"I don't get it... Him?!"*

Sure, her affair partner may not be gainfully employed, may live in his parents' basement, may drive a shitty car, and may have a criminal record... but he's fun, interesting, and something about him pushes her buttons. He makes her feel sexy. He taps into something that makes her "feel alive" again. He allows her to temporarily strip herself of the boring veneer of "wife" and "mom".

The societal pressure is miraculously lifted from her shoulders, one orgasm at a time.

He's her lover. He is no provider. She knows that. That's precisely what she likes about him.

Next thing you know, she is wiping the marriage scoreboard clean. All those provider points you have earned over the years mean exactly zero when somebody comes along and pushes those oft-neglected "time to have sex" buttons of hers.

Men who are left by their wives start listing all the wonderful things they did as provider for her and the family. He's building the case for why her affair is completely irrational.

The wife's reaction: *"Yeah... So?"*

By this point in the relationship, the wife has very real disdain for her husband. Not only is he of no use to her anymore, but he also kept from feeling "so alive" all those years. He wasn't the all-around perfect man she deserved. He was just an obstacle in the way of true happiness and fulfillment. In her mind, this is unforgivable.

The husband is perplexed. This makes no sense.

It's simple: The programming took over.

The Lover wins. Every. Single. Time.

To Be a Good Husband, You Want to be a Good Mix of Lover and Provider

That's what a "real man" is all about. In fact, I will take it a step further and say your scales should be tipped more on the Lover side when in a marriage. You want a good helping of fun, flirty, kinda dangerous, charming, ambitious, sexy tough guy that could bang a pretty woman this week if he wanted to… with a good healthy serving of sweet provider guy thrown in there.

If you're like most guys I chat with, you probably have the provider role down pat. You can do all those great dad/husband things in your sleep. You've probably heard "You're such a good/nice guy" more than a few times your life. Because of your childhood baggage, you may even have real shame and disgust tied to the more "manly" and "masculine" Lover side of you. You may have an untapped wealth of skills and natural ability that you aren't even aware of.

It's time to dive into your Lover side and turn that knob up to eleven. It's been stuck at zero for far too long.

You may surprise yourself with the results.

Be Her Lover - Step #1: Go to the Gym

The lover, more often than not, is a good-looking dude. Not always, of course, but usually. Contrary to popular belief, "good looks" is not a subjective thing. People know "handsome" and "beautiful" when they see it.

Conversely, we also know ugly when we see it.

Science can break down what makes a man "attractive" to women across all cultures, and the "attractive" traits always point to two things:

1. **Health** – nice teeth, clear skin, high energy, positive attitude

2. **High levels of testosterone** – good musculature, good posture, confidence, aggression

Look good. Look healthy. Be active. Be masculine. That about covers it. Not so hard, right? Well, some things can very easily get in the way of attaining your "be attractive" goals as a man.

Comfort is thy enemy.

When men enter a long-term monogamous relationship, it's like a warm and intoxicating bath after a hard day's work. You just settle in, relax, and get comfortable. "Aaaaaah."

No more dating. No more rejection. No more stupid games. No more of all that annoying single life bullshit. Now you can live a "normal" life.

But, of course, there's a tradeoff. With the comfort of a steady and secure relationship comes a slew of negative repercussions. The first and most obvious is the breakdown of your physical appearance. **To put it bluntly, once you say "I do", men tend to get fat and out of shape, and so does the wife.**

You just stop caring about the "shallow" stuff and focus on the more "important" stuff, like paying bills and coaching Billy's soccer team. Men will often point to their busy jobs, kids, and housework as reasons to neglect their appearance and health.

"I would totally go to the gym, but who has the time for that?"

The reality is that it is VERY easy to skip the hard stuff that you really don't HAVE to do. Read more books? Go to the gym? Eat right? Tough habits to keep up. They take time... and spare time is something that people today have very little of, right?

Bullshit.

Sorry, I'm not buying it. You're just being lazy.

I have three kids and I work full-time. More than full-time. My wife works full-time. We travel. I manage to go to the gym 5 days a week. In addition to the gym, I now do stretches and a little light yoga at home before bed. I don't eat like shit. My wife is a busy MD who just recently had not one but TWO serious back surgeries. She was completely incapacitated for a month and is still recovering five months later. She is back in the gym. She still views working on her body as being a habit. There's no question that she has to do it. She's a doctor, she knows how quickly the body can go south if you don't take care of it.

Are you too busy taking kids all over the place? Soccer, basketball, football, boy scouts, etc.? Here's a novel idea: **Stop trying to impress everyone with how many clubs and sports your kids attend.** It's okay if they don't do every activity under the sun. Yes, they can be at home learning how to entertain themselves. They can play with kids in the neighborhood (novel idea). If they must attend that underwater fencing class that is so damn important, arrange for them to go with friends. It's ok for you to not tag along for every single little event.

Take care of yourself for once. There's nothing wrong with trying to be a better and more healthy man.

Let's be honest. Getting in shape is not that hard. We're not talking about building a new addition onto the house.

We're talking about exercise and eating right.

I just would love to eat pizza, drink bourbon and watch football all day... but I can't. I have three kids to feed. Bills to pay. I have a body to maintain. My fitness is right up there with brushing teeth and taking showers. It's just something I do. It's a habit.

Bad habits can get in the way of good ones. Eliminate them. Today. You know what they are. Watching stupid braindead television shows, porn, over-eating... We all know they're not good for us. Be honest with yourself. Be a fucking man and cut them out of your life.

Working out is not hugely time consuming. It's one hour a day. One stupid little hour.

That one hour can transform you into a MUCH healthier and more energetic man. You will add GOOD years to your life. If that's not reason enough... you will LOOK a lot better, and subsequently:

Your wife will be more attracted to you.

Other women will be more attracted to you.

Your wife will notice the other women being more attracted to you and she will become even MORE attracted to you (don't laugh... it's true).

You will be less stressed. You will have more positive energy. This will result in less emoting to your wife.

Men will respect you more.

Your wife will notice men respecting you more and she will become EVEN MORE attracted to you.

Your chances of getting sex from your wife will go up exponentially. Seriously.

"You don't know my wife, dude. Getting abs won't change anything."

Really? Have you tried? I didn't think so.

"But I shouldn't HAVE to go to the gym! She should just want ME for ME!"

For some men, just the thought of having to get fit to impress their wife is insulting. SHE doesn't look that great, after all, and HE still wants HER! Why can't she just suck it up and do the same?

If you find yourself saying this, you have some serious issues you need to work out. You have issues around your perception of reality. You are, again, the stomping spoiled brat who doesn't get his way. Stop thinking about how things SHOULD be. In fact, eliminate the concept of SHOULD from your vocabulary completely. Seriously. It's done nothing but amplify your victim mentality and it makes you unattractive to everyone around you.

Hey, I'm sorry if somebody sold you on the romantic notion

of your wife being sexually aroused by WHO you are and not WHAT you are, but it's just not the complete truth. Yes, your wife loves you for YOU, but as I will say again and again in this book to the point of annoyance... your good-natured ways and track record of awesome dad behavior doesn't push her "must have sex" buttons.

What does help push her buttons are a flat stomach, strong pecs, a nice butt, and powerful arms.

"But my wife says she's not into muscles. She likes nerdy sweet guys."

We are going to keep coming back to the whole concept of "My wife says..." in this book.

Don't listen to her. Watch her actions, instead.

What comes out of her mouth is what she believes you and society want to her to say. In her mind, saying she likes muscles will both hurt your feelings (because...well... look at you) and it will also paint her as some kind of shallow, basic simpleton.

"Wait... you like MUSCLES on a guy? What kind of dumb slut are you?"

If she says she's into nerdy, sweet nice guys, well then society will praise her.

"Oh, you have a deeper and more developed sense of what

is truly attractive in men! Good job, thoughtful lady!"

Trust me, women like masculinity, confidence, and power. Think Fifty Shades of Grey. Think every cover of every romance novel ever made.

What says masculinity, confidence and power more overtly than a muscular and strong physique?

Since I became more muscular, I can tell you that being in shape is an instant button pusher for many women, regardless of their age or background. The muscles give the ladies an excuse to act a little more open and sexual than they normally would. They feel safer doing so. Their preoccupation with what their social circle thinks goes right out the window. It's as if all ladies just inherently understand the situation. It's like they all passed out a memo to each other that read, ***"Control yourself and your sexuality. Don't act slutty. That's not a good thing. Unless, of course, if you're presented with some hunky bombshell of a man. Then you can act like a total moron."***

Ever see footage of a group of women at a bachelorette party with a male stripper? It's insanity. Once the women in the party realize it's ok to act overtly sexual… all bets are off. It can be nothing short of total debauchery. Ironically, it's the complete opposite of a male strip club where the guys all sit like statues and sip their drinks while staring at the naked women. The men don't want to be seen as some kind of creepy perv and thrown out of the place.

The women at the bachelorette party, on the other hand: *"Yes! I get to be a creepy perve! This is fun!"*

Oh, the wonderful and confusing animal that is the human being.

For a myriad of reasons, women will often bottle up their sexuality. They can be a sexual volcano just waiting to blow (pun intended). They just need a good reason to do so and the comfort to know they won't be judged for it.

Have you ever had a woman coworker come up to you and squeeze your arm and say "Nice, Hercules!" or a lady say, "Somebody works out" as she touches your chest? How about a woman lifting your shirt tail to check out your butt?

They're not saying, "I would leave this room and bang you right now", necessarily, but they are saying, *"Congrats. You pushed a button. You made me do something a little silly and risky. Thanks for that, Mr. Muscles. That was fun."*

All of the above happened to me right away after I lost body fat and gained muscle.

"But, dude... my wife HATES muscular athlete type of guys. She says they all look so stupid."

Don't listen to the woman who keeps denying you sex. That's like asking a deer how best to hunt it down and kill it.

"Oh no... keep doing what you're doing! Use that slingshot

and that little rock. That's the best way to take me down, by far. Now if you'll excuse me, I'm going to run away very fast in a zigzag pattern so you can't possibly hit me. Good luck!"

Instead, ask the successful hunter with 50 deer heads on his wall.

"You get a 12-gauge shotgun and you shoot them from close range."

Find a guy who gets lots of sex from his attractive woman (or multiple women) and get his advice. I'll save you some time. You know what they say first and foremost? "Hit the gym." They know the mating game is shallow and stupid. They know how much their life changed for the better when they could finally fill out a t-shirt (in a good way).

The guys at the gym get way more tail than you do. Trust me.

I recognize that there is some pressure amongst your peers to be a fat lazy slob like they are. I see that every day. I'm in my 40's and I'm one of the oldest guys in the gym. That is just sad. I'm not a senior citizen!

Most men my age use golf as their main form of exercise. Most of them look like golf balls themselves. Round, white and covered in dimples.

I remember when I asked some fellow dads if they wanted

to get together to play basketball at the open gym in town. NOPE. No time. They have kid stuff to do. Work is too busy. Blah blah blah.

Meanwhile they are playing fantasy football, golfing, watching sports on TV, eating and, of course, complaining about their pitiful sex lives.

Sad.

They'd rather shove unhealthy food in their faces while watching other men do athletic things. What they don't see is their wife sitting behind them lusting after those football players on TV. She thinks they look really good in their tight pants.

I ended up going to that open gym alone that day. It was me and 7 other guys there. I would say the average age was 19. I hurt for a week after playing just 4 pickup basketball games. It was awesome.

Do things that set you apart from the crowd.

Remember, the goal is for her to be able to point at you from across the room and proudly say, ***"That's MY man right there."***

Your "dad bod" doesn't cut it. It's called a "dad bod" for a reason. All dads have it. It's boring. It's typical. You look like a salamander. You're a cliché. A joke amongst women.

Your dad bod screams comfort. It screams, "I ain't going anywhere". Not because you are faithful and reliable, mind you, but because you CAN'T go anywhere. No other woman lusts after you. That's precisely why women SAY they like dad bods. It gives them a sense of comfort and it makes them feel better about their own lazy and aging bodies. Yes, many women do claim to absolutely LOVE the dad bod. When questioned as to what makes the dad bod so attractive, they will often say, "I can't have a guy that looks better than me. That's just wrong." Translation: ***"If my man was super hot, I would constantly worry about every other woman salivating over him. I have to be assured that I'm not going to lose my mate."***

The dad bod may make them feel more comfortable about themselves, but it doesn't make them want you sexually. There's a huge difference between the two states of mind.

Remember: **If no other woman wants you, then your wife probably doesn't want you, either.**

After you get in shape, other men will notice you being different from the pack (attractive) right away. They may try to avoid you. When you do chat, they will be more submissive. When their wife is around, they will be more aggressive and protective. You will hear men saying things to make you look weaker and inferior around their wives. Their wives aren't stupid. They will pick up on this right away. The man's stupid "mate guarding" tactics backfire. It will end up just making you look more attractive.

You want to be the kind of guy that other men feel nervous leaving their wife alone with.

You'll discover that your newfound muscularity will make your wife nervous and worried. You'll notice more jealousy pop up here and there. She may even get angry at your new fitness hobby. She may have a genuine hissy fit about it. Things are changing and she doesn't like it. She is not at ease.

THIS IS A GOOD THING. DON'T FIGHT IT. STAY THE COURSE.

Welcome to being an attractive dude. It comes with drama.

A lot of men make a mistake at this point. They freak out when their wives get stressed and angry about their positive changes. Then they explain everything away. They tell their wife how they wanted to turn their sex life around so they started going to the gym.

"No no, mommy. Please don't be mad! I was just trying to do things for YOU!"

WRONG WRONG WRONG.

Your newfound level of muscularity and confidence is NOT just for her and your sex life, but for YOU. If you even hint at this being for HER and that you're just trying to improve your sex life, you will go from being sexy to pitiful in a nanosecond.

You're still the nice but creepy guy doing things for affection.

Your self-improvement is for your SELF. The consequences of your self-improvement MAY be more sex from your wife, but sex should never be the overt intention. It sounds stupid… but your woman wants a natural, not a guy who tries out different things to win her love and affection again.

What's the difference between you and a natural? There is none. There's no such thing as a natural. Everyone learns. Whether you are a "natural" or not is all about their perception. If you do something with little effort and do it with no ulterior motive or attention-seeking in mind, you are a "natural".

You just keep taking care of yourself, look better and get healthier. No explaining. No rationalizing. No approval-seeking. Make it a natural, normal part of your life.

Going to the gym, lifting weights, gaining muscle and losing fat is the first step towards turning things around. It's the first and probably the most impactful step. For some men, they can stop right here, and their bedroom situation improves tremendously.

Just watch. Your hard work will inspire your wife to get HER ass back in the gym, too. It's funny how that works.

Couples that are completely mismatched in attraction levels are rare. Unless, of course, we're talking about the super provider man and the trophy wife. We all know about that couple and how that ends.

Think about it. How many times have you seen a super handsome guy with a homely, overweight wife? Exactly.

Your wife knows that is not a sustainable relationship dynamic. Watch her as she instinctively kicks up her own fitness a few notches and starts pointing out her improvements.

"I think my belly looks a little smaller. Don't you?"

She knows she must compete with a lot more women now.

This is a very good thing. Don't you dare go and try and out-nice this instinctive reaction. Believe it or not, your wife is enjoying this new change. She enjoys having to play catch-up to her husband who seems to be hell bent on getting in amazing shape. She actually LIKES that little bit of anxiety and pressure that she's experiencing. It's been a long time since she's looked up to you in this way.

Enjoy it.

Be Her Lover - Step #2: Go Away

The Lover is scarce. He has other things to do. What things? Well, that's not too clear. He may be working hard, doing some hobby, or going out with friends… or possibly out seeing other women.

He's not always available for a quick chat. He doesn't always divulge his whereabouts or plans.

He has a date with his girl planned for Saturday, and he will see her then. She may not hear a peep from him until then.

This drives his women crazy. This is a good thing.

Part of the libido-sucking nature of a long-term monogamous relationship is tied to familiarity and comfort. You can call it "relationship fatigue".

"Oh… it's you again. Great."

You're always there. Your dependable. She just has to say "Honey?!" and you'll be by her side in a nanosecond.

This may sound like what a true "life partner" is supposed to be, but it absolutely kills the female sex drive.

"Familiarity breeds contempt."

"Absence makes the heart grow fonder."

Heard these before? Of course you have.

The natural progression of a typical long-term monogamous relationship includes the initial honeymoon phase, then the fun awkwardness of learning about each other's quirks, blemishes, and vices, and then the stress and boredom as you concentrate on keeping the household/parenting machine running.

As the relationship timeline progresses, the time spent together increases. It's no coincidence that the frequency of sex also goes down at this phase.

Simply put, you need to frequently get away from your wife. You need time for YOU.

Get active. When you are on the couch day after day, your wife's inner cavewoman programming says, "Aren't you supposed to be out chasing sabre tooth tigers and getting us some food or something?" Be energetic. Take on life. Don't let life beat you down and wear you out so easily. Get out there and tackle the world.

Trust me, as a father of three that works full time, I totally understand the desire to just say "fuck it" and relax at home. It's perfectly ok to take a timeout on a regular basis to recalibrate, but it's not ok to do this day after day after day.

Get away from your wife. Go do things for YOU.

Yes, being away from her may increase her anxiety and

cause some worry. But that's ok. Your initial dating life, the "honeymoon phase", was fraught with such anxiety.

Does he like me?
Does he not like me?
Is he tired of me already?
Am I too fat?
Does he respect me?
Oh my god, did I really just say that?
Does this outfit look too slutty?
Does he think I'm stupid?
Is he dating other girls?
Did that girl just look at him? Did he look back? Does he know her?

It sounds exhausting and torturous (welcome to the world of the female mind), but here's what's interesting: That anxiety is a crucial ingredient for what sparked her early relationship libido in the first place.

It's sounds counterintuitive, but these feelings she had weren't necessarily a bad thing. It means she cared and was invested in growing your relationship. **SHE WAS TURNED ON.** She was in the beginning stages of being "in love".

The opposite of being in love is not hate, it's indifference.

When you see each other day after day that anxiety is gone. The drama is gone. She becomes indifferent. She's bored.

NEVER EVER LET YOUR WIFE GET BORED.

Nothing good comes from a bored wife. Ever. She will seek excitement elsewhere.

Drama. Anxiety. Feelings. Excitement. These are the foundation of the female libido. Combine your new high levels of physical fitness with scarcity... and oh boy. Watch out. Drama City, USA.

Embrace the drama and anxiety. Don't run from it. Drama is your friend. It means you're doing something right.

It's okay for her to be a little anxious. Stop trying to alleviate her stress all the time, especially when that stress is indicative of a normal and healthy male-female relationship.

Stop fearing her negativity. Stop with the ***"Ok ok ok... I'll do whatever you want, just stop being a bitch"*** attitude you've had all these years. Your wife wants a man who can take her drama and laugh it off. Remember, the myth of "happy wife = happy life"? Stop tip toeing around her. Let her be anxious and upset.

REMEMBER THIS: YOU'RE DOING NOTHING WRONG.

You're simply getting out of the house and taking care of yourself. You're trying to better yourself as a man. Bravo to you.

Do you have any "player" type of friends that are dating lots of women? Ask them about female drama. Sit back in awe as he shares crazy story after crazy story.

The player gets frequent sex. With sex comes drama. With drama comes sex. He's well aware of this dynamic. He doesn't care. He has a harem of seven different girls he can call on for fun. When Sally gets a little too crazy, he ignores her and calls Debra instead. All the women know about each other. This causes more drama… and consequently more sex for him.

Sounds exhausting, doesn't it? Luckily you have just one drama queen to contend with.

You need time to yourself, even if/when it results in anxiety and drama from your wife. Not only is getting away from her an admittedly manipulative ploy to get your wife's anxiety/libido engine going (more on manipulation later), but it's also mentally healthy for you. You need to discover more of yourself again.

REMEMBER: Things that make you a better man = Things that make your wife horny.

You can't become a better dude if you are constantly by your wife's side. She doesn't hold all the tools to make you a more complete man. Yes, she's your partner and mom to your kid, but she's also a girl. Girls and boys don't do well after being together for long periods of time, in case you didn't notice.

No, hiding in your "man cave" doesn't count. That's just your little designated area of the house. You're still in the house and still with her. You need to get out and do your own thing. Get away from her.

Trust me, she doesn't need you around all the time. She's a big girl and can take care of things for a little while.

Men should welcome the idea of going out on their own. It should be a relief. You should look forward to it. My dad used to go to the hardware store for four hours at a time. He wasn't buying anything (because who really needs to be at the hardware store for FOUR HOURS?!). He was drinking coffee, eating popcorn and "shooting the shit with the boys" while looking at tools and planning his next home project. He needed the time away to recalibrate after being around a kid and wife for so many hours a day.

This is normal and healthy behavior for a man.

NOTE: At the time of this writing, we are enduring a global pandemic. This has resulted in a lot of emails from readers asking, *"How the hell can I GET AWAY now?!"* Ideally, yes, you want to physically remove yourself from the family home. In light of the current situation, the only viable alternative is to mentally escape. Going to a room alone and telling everyone, *"Leave dad alone for a couple of hours"* is perfectly fine. You can use that time to read, listen to audiobooks, podcasts, meditate, plan your next entrepreneurial venture, work on a hobby… anything that removes you mentally from "dad and husband" mode and improves yourself as a man.

I started a new members-only area of my website called **"DSO Fraternity"** that you may find helpful. There are member-only articles, audio, access to all of my books, access to private Facebook groups, and live Zoom meetings where men can get together and talk about their issues. Connecting to other men with the goal of self-improvement is an excellent way to supercharge your efforts. You will reach your end goals A LOT faster by learning from others who have been there and done that before. You can give it a try for $9.99 per month. Cancel anytime. A portion of your membership fee also goes to the Movember Foundation – an excellent charity for men. Check it out at **dadstartingover.com/join.**

Be Her Lover - Step #2: Go Away

For every man, I recommend that you get a "Mission" in life. You need to set a goal or a series of goals. You need a purpose in life outside of your family. You need to create a series of steps to reach that goal. You do those steps a little at a time. Along the way of reaching your goal, you attain little "quick wins" that give your brain and body the boost it needs to keep going. After much hard work and determination, you reach the end goal, only to find that another goal immediately appears in the distance.

This is called being a "man on a mission".

I can't stress enough how important this is. **I can't stress enough how this MUST be something that is geared towards YOU and your interests and falls outside of the realm of the family.** In other words, "I'm going to coach my kid's baseball team to a championship" is not a mission. "I'm going to save up money and take my family to Hawaii" is not a mission.

These are examples of missions:

"I've always wanted to pursue art and sculpting more. I'm going to take classes at the nearby art school. I'm going to mentor with somebody and learn. I'm going to attend my first art show. I'm going to sell my first piece. I'm going to be in the big art gallery in town. Eventually, people all over the world will buy my sculptures through my website."

"I'm going to start a charity for homeless veterans in my city. I'm going to contact some other homeless veteran

charities in other cities to see what it is they are doing to combat the problem. I'm going to learn all I can about mental health. I'm going to talk to struggling veterans to get an idea of what life is like for them. I'm going to put a plan down on paper. I'm going to learn about fundraising. I'm going to open a shelter for homeless veterans in my city... maybe in other cities, as well."

"I'm going to get in the best shape of my life and start a website chronicling my journey. I'm going to learn all I can about diet and exercise and share my results along the way. I'm going to interview experts in the field like doctors and trainers. I'm going to start a podcast about my journey. I'm eventually going to have companies ask to sponsor my site and podcast. I'm going to make this a legitimate second source of income. I'm going to look like a male fitness model and be an inspiration to millions of other normal guys who want to do the same."

When men have a very real mission for life, the act of "getting away" and doing what they can to better themselves as men... that kind of takes care of itself. You'll find yourself hanging out and learning from a growing group of new people that you call friends. You find that you're not so caught up in the day-to-day emotions of your wife, and therefore you're not so needy at home. You'll find, for once, that your wife is the one fighting for YOUR attention and affection. This is normal. This is the dynamic that a woman is typically more comfortable in.

Your wife wants to be in the position of having to earn the

attention and affection from a man on a mission. She wants to tell people that her guy is "just so busy" doing cool and important things. When you and your wife do get together for alone time, it should be an event. It should be fun and sexy break from the domestic life that does such a good job of smothering sexuality and desire.

Get out. Do things. Be a better and more rounded man. Your wife, and your life in general, will thank you.

Be Her Lover - Step #3: Be Unique

In every romantic relationship, we want to believe that the person we picked is different from the rest of the pack. We want to believe that our partner possesses a unique unicorn level of awesomeness that cannot be equaled by anyone else. We want to believe they are extremely scarce and in high demand.

Conversely, you want to portray to your partner that yes, they made the right choice in picking you, as well. You are also a rare find amongst a giant population of losers.

"I'm not like other women." Every woman in a relationship has said this. Every single one. They know how important it is to stray from the pack if they want to achieve peak attractiveness. They know what nutcases many women are and how unattractive that is.

"I'm not like other women… I like hanging out with guys more" is another common statement women give. They feel it gives them a leg up over the competition. Makes them more trust-worthy. It actually does the opposite (a woman who hangs out mostly with men is a relationship red flag).

SIDE NOTE: Many men emailed me after reading the statement above, asking me to expand on this further (apparently a lot of men have heard the "I like hanging out with guys more" line from their wives). As with all red flags, this doesn't necessarily signify "DANGER - YOU'RE WIFE IS CHEATING ON YOU". It just means that it is something to be aware of and to watch carefully. To quote from my third book, "RED FLAGS":

"I just like hanging out with guys more. They're way less drama."

We've all heard this a time or two in our lives. Loosely translated, this means, **"The attention I get from the opposite sex makes me feel special. The fact that I can manipulate and dominate a relationship via my sexuality is a very good thing for me. These types of relationships always work in my favor. Strictly platonic relationships where there is no implied sexuality or exchange of favors is of no use to me. I just feel inadequate when I am in a relationship with equals."**

Ask a woman about the man she's in love with and she will jump immediately into what sets him apart from the rest. She may mention his job and that he's a really sweet guy... but not until she gets out of the way exactly WHY she devotes so much energy to this guy.

"He's really cute. He's into art. He does his own sculptures out of glass and wood. He also plays in a band on some weekends."

You need to stick out from the rest of the pack. Don't blend in. Don't follow the standard script that so many other dads do. Don't be the mopey, boring, dad bod, no style, watch football, take kids to soccer, take out the trash, go to bed, go to work kinda guy. If you just sit back, watch and emulate what everybody else does, you'll just end up getting what everybody else gets: a boring, non-sexual relationship.

Be interesting. Be different.

Uniqueness is an important ingredient for her delicate sex drive soufflé. She craves different. She craves special. She craves unique.

The same ol' same ol' is BORING. Remember: Don't let your wife get bored!

Let's look at this from a more scientific angle:

For a woman to devote herself to YOU and just YOU is a really big deal for her. She does not take it lightly. Ideally, she wants to pick one REALLY GOOD man to stick with for a long time.

Because… what if she gets pregnant? She's then stuck with this guy and his offspring for YEARS.

This man she has chosen better be healthy, smart, tough… an all-around good dude. Not only does he need to pass on his great healthy man genes to the baby, but he also needs to stick around to help take care of her and the kid.

Remember: Lover + Provider = Ideal man

If he's not that kind of guy, then she has made a giant life-changing mistake. Unfortunately, most guys are NOT that kind of guy. At all. Ask any woman who has been single for a while. It's scary how bad their male pool of candidates is.

Therefore, the kind of guy they want is "different" from the rest of that pitiful pack of candidates out there.

When her brain feels, "He's different and worthy of my attention", that's a crucial step towards turning the sexual engine on.

"I don't know why, but I like you."

Why do you think the skinny, androgynous rock star makes women so weak in the knees? He's literally UP ON THE PEDESTAL of the stage, away from the rest of the plebes. Lights are shining on him. He's the most important person in the building at that moment. He's confident. He looks like a total weirdo, but he doesn't care. Everyone can see him. Everyone can hear him. He can do whatever and their eyes will follow.

Women stare in awe, put their hands to the face and scream. It's all just too much to take in.

The rock star is about as different, unique, interesting and stand-out-from-the-pack as you can get. It's not about his money, either. Ask any single guy who started up a garage band and started doing gigs for $500 on weekends. He rarely went back home without a girl on his arm. It's like shooting fish in a barrel for him.

Him: *"I play guitar for the band."*

Her: *"Oh, reeeeaaally? That's so awesome!" (twirling her hair)*

To further illustrate the importance of being unique, are you familiar with the world of "Pickup Artists"? It's a hilarious and extremely interesting sub-culture of socially awkward men (dorks) who discovered that their success rate of "picking up" women can be dramatically improved by doing and saying very specific things at just the right time.

They're basically some nerds that studied women like lab rats and watched how they behave in certain conditions. They see what actions create interest and which don't. They see which actions result in getting the woman's number and which actions result in getting ignored or a drink thrown in their face.

Obviously, the pickup artist is not too popular with women or society in general. Nobody likes being treated like lab rats. Nobody likes a fraud who learned how to fake being charming. We all like "naturals".

With that being said, a lot of what the pickup artists teach actually works. It's sometimes forced, contrived and completely cringe-worthy, but if they do everything right, they achieve their goal: they get laid way more often than they did before. All morals aside, that's a win in their book.

One important concept the pickup artists push is called

"peacocking". Picture a male peacock fanning his feathers open and strutting around in front of a female. He's saying, "Does this bountiful and colorful plumage set me apart from the rest? I have some GOOD genes here, girlfriend. I make very healthy babies."

Peacocking is the same in humans. You must visually set yourself apart from the pack. You could be a muscular Adonis with a chiseled jaw and pecs bulging out of your shirt… or you could wear something flamboyant and ridiculous that makes women stop and go "What the…?" It may be a leopard print coat, a giant fuzzy hat, painted nails… whatever. It's admittedly ridiculous, but all this peacocking has a purpose. It says:

"I'm unique. Plus, I really don't give a shit what other people think about me. That makes me doubly unique."

I don't recommend walking around with a toilet plunger stuck to your head and a glowing set of pink nipple rings while at home with your wife… but the underlying concept is valid. Stick out somehow. Don't give a shit what everyone else thinks. Don't be needy. Don't be anxious. Be unique.

Do something that makes her say, "Yep… I picked a good one. He's different than the rest of you assholes."

Some ideas:

1. Take a dance class.
2. Take up a form of art like painting, sculpting or

photography.
3. Learn a martial art, like Jiu Jitsu.
4. Coach your kid's sport team.
5. Start up a charity.
6. Write a book.
7. Play an instrument.
8. Take an acting class.

At this point in the book, what should start to click in your brain now is that all of this is not a "trick". It's not "manipulation". It's work. It's called, "being a better man". As I say in my book "NOW WHAT?", it's called being a **Mentally Healthy Non-Needy Man (MHNNM)**.

Remember: **Things that make you a better man, are things that make your woman horny for you.**

Be Her Lover - Step #4: You Must Lead and Set the Tone of the Relationship

A guy reaches out to me and complains about lack of sex with his wife. He gives the typical list of provider traits as proof of his worth: He works hard, he's a great dad, he buys things for his wife, he has been faithful (even though he had some easy opportunities to cheat in the past – all men point this out to me for some reason), he doesn't flirt with other women, he helps around the house and with the kids a lot, etc.

Me: *"Okay... but what do you do that is SEXY?"*

Him: *"What do you mean?"*

Me: *"You know... what do you do to set the mood? How do you let her know you love her, find her attractive, and want her sexually?"*

Him: *"I tell her."*

Me: *"What do you tell her?"*

Him: *"That I love her."*

Me: *"Well... You tell your kids you love them. That's not sexy. How do you go from that to sexy?"*

Him: *"I'll give her massages and stuff when we go to bed sometimes. She really likes that. Then I ask her if she feels like having sex. She usually says no. I don't know what else to do. Oh, and sometimes we go out to dinner just the two of us, when my parents can watch the kids. Go to the movies... stuff like that."*

Wow... how does she keep her hands off of you, casa nova?

This is so very typical for men. Guys thinking like guys. They think it's a 4-step process.

1. Lay down next to wife.
2. Give her a massage or an overt sexual signal (like grabbing her boob).
3. Say you love her.
4. Ask for sex.

No.

Remember... **delicate soufflé.** This isn't a firecracker you just light and watch explode. This is a recipe that has lots of ingredients. Baking this soufflé takes TIME. Patience.

It is up to you to set the tone of sexiness in the relationship. If you sit back and wait for your wife to initiate sex without ANY action on your part, you will be one frustrated dude. I don't mean massaging her and saying, "Let's fuck", I mean being way more subtle, genuine, and consistent over a longer period of time.

Here are some examples of small actions you can do over the next few months to set the proper tone (NOTE: These ideas will only work if you have your physicality and mindset in line. Do all of the other steps first):

When you walk by your wife at home, give her a little brush and squeeze with your hand. Just a little something to say "I'm here… I see you there, sexy girl. I appreciate you." Nothing more. Just the little squeeze of the arm or shoulder. A hand on the small of her back. No words.

Walking behind her while she cooks? Give her a smooch on the back of her head. Tell her she looks beautiful. Tell her how much you love her. Walk away. Nothing else.

She's carrying a load of laundry? Grab it from her. *"Here babe, I got it."* As you reach for the basket, pull her in and give her a smooch. Say to her, "You look really good today." Leave it at that.

She's getting ready in the morning in front of the bedroom mirror? Give her butt a squeeze and say "Mmmm. That's what I like right there." Walk away. Nothing more.

You're giving little gifts of love and affection. It's part of setting the tone. With those brief little touches and kisses, you're reminding your wife that she's more than just a mom. She's a woman.

You are setting the stage for genuine connection. You are

telling her that you're still a COUPLE and not just mom and dad. You are NOT doing these things because you expect sex. In fact, you don't care if she reciprocates your affection or not. She may be frustrated at times with your touches and bluntly say, *"NO SEX TONIGHT!"* That's cool with you. You just smile and joke with her: "Wow… pervert. Who said anything about sex?" Or a smile, a simple "Ok" and a quick change of topic will do.

Outcome should never be on your mind when it comes to these little signs of connection.

Her little verbal jabs should just bounce right off of you. This is very important and crucial for setting the right tone in the relationship. You don't give two shits if your actions result in sex or not. Your feelings are not so easily hurt. You are not so emotionally dependent upon her reaction to you and what you do.

Note: Little verbal jabs from your wife CAN later become real toxic asshole behavior. Context is everything. If she's being offensive or disrespectful for no damn reason, let her know right then and there. Don't wait. Call her out on it.

You're the man. You love her. You appreciate her. She doesn't want to reciprocate your little positive moments right then and there? Meh… no biggy. You're not doing these things to get mommy's approval. You're doing them because you're a loving, sexual creature. She's a woman. You're a man. You are awesome. These very brief little gifts of attention are reminders of that.

You need to present an aura of, ***"I'm sexy...I love you... here, let me give you a little smooch to remind you of how much you mean to me. Now I need to go do something else. I'm a valuable dude."***

Just like regular gift-giving and chores, you do these little things because you WANT to do them.

You do them from a genuine "I really don't give a shit if you do anything in return or not" mindset.

You're projecting an image of high value, confidence, sexiness, and lustfulness without a hint of neediness or expectation of reward. <- This is extremely important to internalize.

Neediness should never be the foundation of your love and affection. All that neediness does is put more pressure and stress on your wife. Sex with you should not be a chore or a requirement of her as your wife, but instead it should be a natural progression of your already sexual and fun relationship.

With the neediness gone, the pressure is lifted from your wife's shoulders. She suddenly has one less kid in the house. She has a man. A high-value man who still has desire for her even after all these months/years of being neglected.

Combine this loving aloofness with your new gym body,

your independence, and your unique qualities that set you apart from the rest... and eventually she'll start to feel that little twitch in the back of her mind. That's when the brain starts churning away with all those estrogen-fueled thoughts and anxiety.

"What was that about? That was sweet of him. Why did he do that? I should've kissed him back. Does he still expect sex? I really don't feel like it. When's the last time we had sex? I bet he's just doing that for sex. I get tired of his whining. Where's he going? He did that this morning, too. He hasn't asked me for sex in a while. Maybe he found somebody else. No way. Could be... I mean, I saw how that woman at work was flirting with him. I don't even think he noticed... or maybe he did notice and they're having a secret affair and he tried to act all innocent. He has been going to the gym more. He looks better than I do. I bet he thinks I'm gross. I have a horrible mom body. I should go to yoga with Sally. Wait, was that a new shirt he had on? When did he buy that? Maybe his mistress bought it for him. Oh my god... is this a midlife crisis? Suzy's husband left her for that young secretary last year. No way my husband would do that, though. Or would he? That would be so embarrassing for me and terrible for the kids. Everyone will think I was too ugly for him. I bet he's totally cheating. What if he isn't? Am I a terrible wife?"

Exhausting to read, but does it look familiar? This is similar to the anxiety she felt at the beginning of your relationship. This is the little natural twinge of worry that so many guys try to squash immediately. But, you're smart. You're different. You know this is a good thing. This means she's starting to feel attraction towards you again. You let her brain do its thing and you just keep being the best and most attractive guy you can be.

There's nothing you can do to stop her brain from spinning a mile a minute. Nor do you want to.

"But, she's going to think I'm cheating on her!"

And? So what? Are you really cheating on her? NO. You're simply being the awesome guy that so many other women in her shoes would KILL to have at home. That's why she's anxious. It's not because you're doing anything wrong. You're not at all. You're doing everything RIGHT. That puts pressure on her. This reintroduces feelings she hasn't experienced in a quite a while.

You're making progress.

Repeat after me: You're doing nothing wrong.

STOP FEELING SO DAMN SHAMEFUL ABOUT BEING A BETTER MAN.

You're a good dude doing good things to attempt to reignite your wife's desire for you… so that you two can continue staying together in a happy marriage. Just like you promised to do in your vows on your wedding day.

Wow. How horrible. You manipulative monster. How do

you live with yourself?

It's shortly after her brains spins out of control that she will decide to consult with a friend or two about your situation. Here's how a typical friend conversation will go:

Wife: *"I'm worried about Steve. He's not acting right."*

Friend: *"What's going on?"*

Wife: *"I think he's having a midlife crisis."*

Friend: *"Oh no! What's he doing?"*

Wife: *"He lost some weight... started going to the gym. He's dressing all young and sexy now. It's very weird."*

Friend: *"Oh no... that's how Sally's husband acted before he left her and the kids. Remember?"*

Wife: *"Yeah, I know. That's why I'm worried."*

Friend: *"Does he act like he hates you now? Ignores you? Starts fights for no reason?"*

Wife: *"No, he's been very sweet lately. Loving. Gives me kisses all the time. He grabs my butt and stuff more now. Calls me beautiful."*

Friend: *"Oh, well that's great. Maybe he realizes what a catch you are and he's just trying to be better. He sounds like Sara's* husband, Joe. He's great to her. They're probably the happiest couple I know. She just got boob implants last week. She says they were a gift to him... to keep him away from the young girls. Ha! They just went on a cruise last week. You should see their pictures. They both look really good for their age."

Wife: "Yeah, I'm not getting boob implants anytime soon! Maybe I'm overreacting. It makes me realize what a bitch I've been for a while. He's doing all these things... and he doesn't ask anything of me, ever. We also haven't had sex in a while. He stopped pressuring me."

Friend: "Oh really? That's not good. How long has it been since you had sex?"

Wife: "I dunno... weeks? Maybe months?"

Friend: "Oh, sweetie... that's not good. And he's not asking for it? A man can't go on that long without sex. He's going to explode. That's what happened with Sally's husband. They had the baby and she didn't want sex anymore. He got a new girlfriend almost immediately and filed for divorce."

Wife: "I know. Trust me, I get it. It doesn't help that other women are staring at him all the time. He's so clueless he doesn't even notice. He took his shirt off and was showing off his new abs the other day when he washed the car outside in the driveway. I think Karen next door about had a heart attack. Even her husband was staring."

Friend: "Steve has abs now?! Wow. I didn't know that. My

husband hasn't been in good shape since...ever. Good for you, girlfriend! You got a hotty for a husband! You really need to take care of him, then! If you won't, trust me... somebody else will!"

Wife: *"Yeah, I guess. I should probably get my flabby ass back in the gym, then. Haha."*

Friend: *"Yeah. Wow...I mean, no! You look great. I knew Steve was looking really good lately, but didn't know he was in THAT good of shape."*

Wife: *"Alright, don't you start drooling, too! That's my husband we're talking about!"*

Friend: *"I know! You're a lucky girl. It may not last! I'd be enjoying it if I were you."*

Notice how she went from *"I'm worried about his weird behavior"* to *"Yeah, I guess I am lucky and should get my ass in the gym instead of whining"*? You think this conversation sounds made up or far-fetched? Hell no. This is a very realistic example what could happen when your wife starts getting anxious about your changes.

Woman is annoyed and worried about new husband behavior.

She doesn't know quite how to process so she confers with peer group.

Peer group digests information and points out that her husband is attractive to others and loving. This is good and she should shape her ass up.

She agrees to shape her ass up and stop whining about nothing.

A lot of guys, myself included, really don't understand why their wife needs to check in with girlfriends all the time to confirm what is so obvious to everyone else. I used to get REALLY upset with my ex-wife for checking in with her peer group about every little thing I would say or do. For one, I saw it as a lack of respect towards me (it was)... and two, it made me feel less respect for her. What kind of adult needs to check-in with people all the time to form an opinion about things that are so basic?

It could be about the absolute dumbest things:

Me: *"No, sweetie. You don't want to pour that bacon grease down the drain. It can clog the pipes and it's no good for the sewer. Just put it in the trash can."*

Ex-wife: *"No, I'm pretty sure you can pour it down the drain."* *continues pouring down the drain*

Me: *"No, just dump it in the trash. Please."*

NEXT DAY

Ex-wife: *"I talked to Sally at work and she says you shouldn't put bacon grease down the drain."*

Me: *"Oh, good. I'm glad you checked in with Sally, The Queen Chancellor of Bacon Grease, just to make sure. Or you could just listen to your husband for once..."*

You must come to terms with the fact that much of how your wife feels and how she processes things about you and your relationship is largely determined by her peer group. If you do something that pisses her best friend Sally off, you damn well better believe that Sally will let your wife know ASAP and not let up until your wife does something about it.

Conversely, if you do something that Sally thinks is amazing… your wife will also hear about it too. Sally gushing over you will win you A LOT of attraction points. Sally's pushing the buttons for you. That's a very good thing.

The lesson: **Women are very social creatures**. They want both direction and acceptance from their peer group. They want reassurance. Your wife WILL take Sally's advice and perspective to heart and it will affect your marriage. Good or bad. That's just the way it is.

What you want to do is set the tone of the relationship so that it minimizes the impact of stupid negative outside influencers like Sally. You want to become an undeniably good thing. You want to become the guy that repeatedly pushes her buttons. You want to become the husband that the other wives can't wait to hear stories about. You want your wife to be your number one fan. That is when the wife sees herself as part of your TEAM, rather than the stressed-out wife who constantly complains about her husband. When she's part of your team, it's you two against the rest of the world.

That's when you do your best as a couple. That's when your wife will be the happiest… as your co-captain in life.

Get Her Away From The Kids

As I have said many times in my writing, parenthood is the antithesis of eroticism. The two worlds do not mesh. As far as "major turnoffs" are concerned, being a parent is right up around the top of the list (along with global pandemics, job loss, and farting husbands). When your wife is in MOM mode, she is ONLY in mom mode.

Many men make the mistake of trying to introduce overt sexuality into situations where it just doesn't belong:

The wife is busy wiping up baby vomit and the husband reaches down and gives her dangling sore mom boob a squeeze. He seems genuinely perplexed and hurt when she yells, *"CAN YOU PLEASE NOT DO THAT?!"*

The wife just finished yelling at the 15-year-old for the hundredth time about stupid things the dumb teen keeps insisting on doing. The wife looks like she has been to hell and back. Dad looks at his wife sympathetically and says, *"So… you wanna do it tonight? We didn't get around to doing it last week like we said we would."* She turns around and goes into the other room without saying a word.

Mom got a call from the school. The 9-year-old got into a fight at and broke the other kid's nose. The wife is very upset. She sobs and says that she can't believe her son is a "bully" and would do something like that. Husband assures her that it is no big deal, boys fight sometimes, and besides, *"I'll make you feel all better tonight in the bathtub."* The wife immediately looks up at the husband with tears streaming down her face. *"What the fuck is*

wrong with you?"

When it comes to getting your wife in the right headspace for sexuality, it's all about CONTEXT. Simply put, having children is a short-cut method to ruining your sex life. I can't tell you how many men have told me that sex with their wife ceased after their new baby came into the world. The wife's body and brain just shifted gears completely. **"MOM MODE: ENGAGED. MUST PROTECT BABY. EVERYTHING ELSE COMES SECOND TO BABY. IGNORE HUSBAND."**

Many men believe that this was an evil and manipulative bait and switch routine on the part of the wife. She just needed him to procreate. Once the baby came out, she was free to shut down the sex life that she was never really into to begin with. I'm sure that happens from time to time, but the more realistic and less sinister truth is that she USED to want intimacy with her husband, but under the pressure of being a new parent, the world of sexuality is completely smothered. What used to come "naturally" now takes "work"… and as any parent will tell you, **adding more "work" to your to-do list sounds like the last thing you want to do.**

For MANY couples, if you want to grow closer together and increase your chances of intimacy, you need to get away from the world of parenthood as much as humanly possible. Do so on a regular basis. Date nights are a must, but that is the minimum. You need weekends away. You need to leave the kids with grandma and grandpa, aunts and uncles,

146

friends… and go away together on an adventure as a couple.

I always recommend to men that they plan a surprise trip without telling the wife about any of the details. Arrange all of the logistics needed to make the trip happen. Arrange for childcare. Plan the trip. Pay for everything up front. Play the part of the leader. Your wife should come home from work and see a husband sitting on the couch with a suitcase next to him.

You: *"Welcome home, beautiful. You have one hour to get ready. You and I are going on a trip. Bring a bathing suit, one nice dress for going out for dinner, and lots of casual clothes for hiking. We will be gone for three days. Everything is planned for and taken care of."*

Her: *"Uhhhh… what? What about the kids? Billy has baseball tomorrow and I have to work on that project with Sally. Remember?"*

You: *"As I said, all taken care of. The kids are handled. Trust me. Everything has been planned. All you have to worry about is relaxing and enjoying a fun trip with your husband. Now, I suggest you hurry… you have 55 minutes left to get ready."*

A lot of men will try some semblance of the "surprise trip" and get angry as their wife throws every protest imaginable at him. "I'm trying to be an awesome husband for her! Why is she such a bitch about it!?" You can think of this reaction from her as a type of shit test. Let it bounce off of you. Of course she is going to protest. Of course she is going to be anxious. You just threw a giant left-turn into her life and disrupted her routine. She's a typical stressed-out mom. On top of that, she probably is not convinced that you can handle such planning without her (because you handed her the reigns of the relationship for so many years). She may have immediately, in her mind, jumped to "Let me imagine the 28 ways that he's going to fuck this up." Plus, if you have been routinely pressuring your wife to have sex with you (the dreaded "talk"), then she probably views this as yet another ploy to get into her pants.

What you do is simple: You plan everything out. You don't let her words bother you. You don't push for sex. You simply enjoy time away from the kids with your wife. **You work on reconnecting as a couple. You allow her to take off her "MOM" uniform and go back to the old, single her… if maybe just for a few days.**

Should You Initiate Sex With Your Wife?

One of the most common questions I receive from readers of the first edition of The Dead Bedroom Fix: ***"Wait... I'm confused. Should I initiate with my wife, or not?"***

Context is everything. Your response to your wife is everything. If you've put in the hard work outlined in this book, and you feel the planets are aligned just right, and you're getting signals from your wife that she is open and relaxed and ready for intimacy, then go ahead and make a move. Be smooth about it. Start slow. Little moves. Back away. More moves. Back away. Make it fun. Make it playful. Don't make it a chore. Don't go full-blown porno star right outta the gate. If she hesitates or acts like she's not ready, back off. No big deal. You're an adult male. You're not a slave to your balls. You're intelligent and mature enough to recognize that your wife isn't there yet. You jumped the gun a little bit. No biggy. We've all done it.

You may find that this new "Hey, this is no big deal" attitude is a GIANT TURN-ON to your wife.

You're not needy. You're a man. James Bond wouldn't jump up and pout and say, "It's not fair! You've been giving me signals all day! We're supposed to have sex!"

Be cool. Baby steps. This stuff takes time.

One Uncomfortable Politically-Incorrect Truth: Women Are Way More Pliable Than You Think

After my wife left, the neighbors on either side of our house divorced. The wives left their husbands. It's true. Do you think that was a coincidence? Nope. The ladies talked. They compared notes. A little story here and a little story there and they are convinced that those little annoying things their husband did over the years weren't so little after all. In fact, they're pretty big and worthy of rethinking this whole marriage thing. The pros outweighed the cons. The women decided they were better off without their men.

Yes, it can be that stupid and drastic. These stories are not unique in any way shape or form.

This is precisely why you keep your wife away from the newly divorced alcoholic gal from the office. This is why you should have a little alarm going off in your head when your wife goes on a "girls' night out" three weeks in a row and leaves you with the kids.

Not only do friends act as major influencers over a woman's day-to-day behavior, but the woman's romantic partner can morph her into a completely new human being, as well. Ever watch a woman who is smitten with a guy completely and totally change her lifestyle and demeanor to match that of her lover? It happens ALL the time.

Women tend to be higher in agreeableness and empathy. This personality traits lead to more "going with the flow" type of actions and a tendency to look for direction and follow the strongest the leader. In general, it makes women the more submissive sex.

Some real-world examples of women who have morphed to take on the traits of their new lover:

A buttoned-up fifty-something conservative grandma and Marketing VP who was single for 12 years (her husband cheated on her) finally dates a man who pushes her buttons. He is a huge Harley Davidson enthusiast and motorcycle club member. She quickly becomes a leather-clad tattooed biker chick with fake boobs. She and her biker boyfriend ride their motorcycles all over the country and they couldn't be happier. She bears zero resemblance to the woman from just a year ago.

A boring, "low libido" forty-something mom of three with a PhD has an affair, divorces her husband, and turns into a tattooed bodybuilding swinger who ignores her children. When she's not participating in orgies or lifting weights, she's routinely on social media proclaiming that she is "the happiest" she's ever been. All her family and friends say she is a completely different human being.

A boring thirty-something housewife and mom of two goes back to school to get her degree. She eventually has sex with three young fraternity guys and divorces husband to be with one of them. She dresses like she's 20

again, gets a nose piercing, colors her hair and ignores her children. The new boyfriend is unemployed and spends his time smoking pot in his parents' basement. The ex-husband has majority custody of the kids. If asked, she will say her ex-husband lied and "stole" the kids from her.

All three of the above scenarios occurred in my extended circle of friends. No, these women are not crazy. They're human beings in love. Their buttons have been pushed. This is probably a new feeling for them. When they're in love, they will morph and change into whatever form they feel is necessary to keep their new man around. The do so unconsciously. The new Lover makes them feel better than they ever have before in their entire life and they don't want to lose that. He is, in essence, a drug that they never want to stop using.

The Lover pushed their buttons and they reacted in a very predictable, albeit drastic way. The programming is in motion. The woman's hindbrain has determined that the Mr. Lover Man is worthy of her time, attention, and her body. If that means taking on a new persona and flushing away her old life, then so be it.

No, I don't live in some crazy secret world of cheaters and insane women. This is real life. I could give you 1,000 other real-world examples from guys all over the country that I have talked to over the past few years as well as the hundreds of thousands of stories online.

All stories end with the same phrase: "This is not my wife."

This is precisely why I contend that it is possible to reignite the passion in your "low libido" wife. Create the right atmosphere, project the right mentality, push the right buttons... and you're off to the races.

You want a slut at home? Make her one.

You be the Leader. She Should Just Come Along for the Ride.

Set the tone. Be genuine. Push the buttons. She will follow.

You're the guy who is going places. You're the one that is interesting, good looking and different from all the other husbands out there.

You're the prize.

If she wants to jump on this awesome train, she better hurry up and do so.

That's the tone of the relationships I mentioned earlier, where the woman morphed into a different person. She naturally saw this guy who, in her little world, was just so different and awesome that she submitted completely to him.

These women didn't just morph into a new lifestyle, pretend to like it and force a smile the whole way. No, they were eager and happy to submit and go along for the ride. It puts them at ease to have a man who has laid out a blueprint for life and fun. One less thing to worry about!

The supreme irony in all this is that all women, if allowed, will default to being the manager of the family unit. She will plan. She will decide. Eventually, she will grow to hate the job. Every year of being the lone planner and decision maker will build her resentment and push her libido further down in the hole.

If your woman is making plans, you damn well better jump to attention. Don't put your hands behind your head, your feet up and say, "Oh nice. I don't have to worry about this. My wife can handle it." You should jump right in, give your opinion, and find out where you can help. In a gradual way, try taking over the management of the task. "Okay, babe. You go do this and this…and I will take care of the other three things."

I have heard more than one woman say, "I would just like for once to not have to make all the decisions about everything. One day I'd like to not have to THINK and just let somebody ELSE do it!" When your wife leads the family and your relationship, the tone is invariably one of frustration and anger. She will grow tired of playing task master and of the man who so easily submits to her rule. She doesn't want to be the leader of the tribe all day ever day.

She gets tired of seeing your clothes on the floor, watching your beer belly grow, watching you whine about lack of sex, seeing you ignore the chores that need to be done (or worse, doing the chores and seeking her approval), and her being the only one to call and arrange for all those important family events.

She wants a man who takes care of things and always looks to improve himself and the family.

She wants an interesting man. She wants a man who is not afraid of saying what he thinks about her or their relationship at any given moment. She wants a man who won't put up with her bullshit.

In short, she wants it all.

She wants to submit to a guy who throws her on the back of the proverbial motorcycle and says, "Hold on" as he weaves through traffic on his way to adventure and parts unknown.

That guy gets laid.

CHAPTER 5
"This is Manipulation"

If you ever find yourself talking about how to be a better man, or more specifically, how to be more successful with women, you will probably hear something like the following:

"That's manipulation. You're being fake."

By bettering yourself physically, getting away from your family to concentrate on yourself, not putting up with your wife's bullshit, and being open with your sexuality... you're being "manipulative"? Seriously?

What people are really saying:

"You're not actually being YOU. We much prefer to see the real YOU, and not some fake guy going through the motions and pretending to be more than what he REALLY is. If you're a true, natural all-around great dude, then that's great. If you're just a weak guy who is pretending and TRYING to be a good all-around dude, then no.... that's not good. We will openly shame you for that."

Remember, people want to associate with "natural" men, not guys who are learning how to be better and more attractive. Of course, the concept of the "natural" is ridiculous. Nobody was born with an innate knowledge of how to be attractive and get laid. They learned by watching others over the years.

Look at who is doing the shaming. Look at who is most vocally against your "manipulative" behavior.

1. **Women.** These are the same women who put on makeup, color their hair, lie about their age, wear spandex leggings to hide their cellulite and lie about the number of men they have slept with.

These same women are concerned about men being "manipulative"? Seriously? Of course. This is their game, not yours.

To be disingenuous in the mating game is accepted as being in the woman's realm, not the man's. The man must present his TRUE self so that the woman doesn't make the mistake of picking the wrong guy. Remember: It's a huge deal for a woman to pick a man. There's a lot riding on her decision (babies, resources, etc.). She can't put up with any bullshit.

The "no manipulation" rule does not apply to her. Manipulation is an essential element of the female dating game. It's up to men to figure out what is real and what isn't. The more in the dark men are, the better.

For the men to play the same manipulation game is just plain creepy.

2. **Weak men**. There is an understood dominance hierarchy amongst men. Get a group of guys together and somebody will invariably come out as the leader. The rest will fall behind. Picture it as a pyramid of power. The powerful are the few at the top, then everyone else at the bottom.

The same applies to the world of relationships. "The top-dog gets all the bitches", as they say. When a man at the bottom of the pyramid watches as the few men at the top get all the sex, he will grow resentful. He still has his overwhelming urge to have sex with as many women as possible, so he does what he can to elbow his way into the top-tier group and stake his claim. That may mean trying to sabotage the efforts of the higher-ranking men (cock-blocking, in other words). That may also mean befriending women with the sneaky purpose of getting sex somewhere down the line (trying to escape the friend-zone).

These men are the true creeps. They are conniving and manipulative to the core.

These men are some of the first to put down your efforts towards self-improvement. Be aware of them, but they should be ignored completely. Their loser mentality is infectious. Remember, their worries never come from a place of true empathy, but rather from a place of competition. They are attempting to sabotage your efforts as a man trying to rise in the hierarchy.

People often put men and women into comfortable categories and roles. ***"You... You're a provider. You... You're a mom. You... You're a slut."*** When you go outside of those little boxes they put you in, people react almost with hostility and disbelief.

This is especially true if you are encroaching in on their own territory.

Watch the needy but sweet guy walk up to the pretty girl at the bar and tell her that she has a great body, or worse… try to touch her. Watch the scantily clad "slutty" girl interview for a position at a daycare center.

The reaction is always the same: Some variation of *"Uhhh… what are YOU doing HERE? Aren't you supposed to be somewhere ELSE? Know your role in life!"*

You may receive the same type of hostile disbelief or anger when you attempt to shed some of your Provider/Pushover/ Nice Guy behaviors in the hopes of earning more Lover points and rewards. You've been playing the same role for YEARS now. People won't know what the hell to think with a radical change in behavior. Some will flat out hate you for it.

This is very troubling to a lot of men. "I'm still the same sweet guy!" they say to their partner and old friends… only to be hated even more. Why? Because you failed their shit test. They actually RESPECTED the new you more than the old you. They poked at you a little to see if the changes were genuine. You folded. Now they know you belong to the group of weak and manipulative men that everyone detests. Remember: You're trying to better yourself and, consequently, improve your marriage with your wife. You're doing nothing wrong. Stay the course. You're making progress. Every person who has experienced a modicum of success will tell you that the phenomenon of people trying to test you and throw you off your mission is VERY common.

Eventually, if you do your job right, they will gladly come along for the ride.

CHAPTER 6
"Holy Shit. It Worked."

"Work hard in silence. Let success make the noise.'"

Anonymous

Your "Eureka!" Moment Has Arrived

It took months of difficult changes on your part… but you finally did it.

You come home one day and there is a text from your wife as soon as you walk in the door. It simply says, "Go to the bedroom". You walk to the bedroom expecting some major disaster requiring your attention. Maybe there is a wasp in the closet again, or the dog took a giant shit on the carpet. You walk down the hall, turn the corner and you're shocked to your find your wife, naked, covered in baby oil, lying on the bed saying, *"It's about time you got home."*

Holy shit. It worked. You pushed the right buttons in the right combination and her sexual engine fired up again.

You did it.

But wait… there's a rub. There's always a rub. You thought it was going to be that easy?

You may not want her anymore.

"Wait, what?! There's no way!" you're saying right now. Yep. This is common. This is the "bad" part of going through major life changes and dramatic self-improvement.

YOU FINALLY RECOGNIZE YOUR WORTH.

This is precisely why your wife was so nervous about your sudden change in behavior. What she knew deep down was true: She may not be able to match your new level of self-improvement. Your vast improvements in physical appearance, confidence and overall attitude have also fully exposed her faults as a romantic partner.

Let's be honest, your wife is no spring chicken anymore. She knows that it is not uncommon for older attractive men to have a girlfriend half their age. She knows she cannot compete with Buffy the hot little 22-year-old at the gym who all the guys drool over. No amount of makeup, boob jobs or time at the gym can turn back the hands of time and allow her to compare favorably to Bimbo Buffy at the most primal and shallow level of "attraction". She's fully aware of this fact. She's seen the porn videos that you were caught looking at. She's seen you unconsciously staring at girls in public. She knows what all of these women have in common. She knows what pushes your buttons.

She also can't magically erase the years of resentment you have built up after going so long without sexual intimacy. She is one nervous and anxious spouse right now, and for good reason.

You're pissed. You're horny. You're a high-value man in a sea of attractive single women. You've been hit on or approached by a few of these ladies over the past few months. Bimbo Buffy at the gym actually said hi and smiled at you the other day. This has never happened to you before. It's exhilarating. These women are pushing your caveman buttons, big time.

If you're being totally honest, these women make your wife look very blah and unattractive. You feel terrible for thinking this way, but there's no way around it. They're hot. Your wife is not. Your wife gave up on trying to win your admiration and affection long ago.

Your dramatic self-improvements have opened a new world for you. A new circle of friends. You're now around people who also take self-improvement to heart. New guy friends. New female admirers. Consequently, your admiration and attraction for your wife has dwindled. Coming home to her just doesn't have the same appeal that it used to. Being around your wife is a major downer.

"Lucky" for you, your wife finally woke up and said, *"Alright… I see all these improvements you've made, Mr. Husband. Now I'm genuinely turned on and I will gladly allow you access to my body. Please come to the bedroom for your reward."*

You had to jump through A LOT of hoops to get to this point. Really tough stuff. Life-altering self-improvement. Sacrifices. She simply had to sit there and flip a switch in her head, get turned on, and finally realize what a great all-around guy she is married to.

It's at this point you may get a great deal of satisfaction by looking at her on the bed and saying, *"Not tonight, honey. I have a headache"* as you walk away and pump your fist like you just hit a homerun in the World Series.

Don't be petty. Don't be a vindictive little bitch. Be a man.

Life presents you with a lot of tests and temptations, and this is one of them. My advice is to be the leader. Show her how things are done. Set aside your ego. This is your time to shine.

Bang the living snot out of that woman.

Take all those frustrations out in the bedroom. Your attitude should be, *"Here, let me show you what you've been missing."* Make sure for the rest of the week she has a big goofy smile on her face and a pronounced limp.

You made vows. You stick to them. You're a man. That's what you do. If all of us jumped ship every time the grass looked greener elsewhere, there would be no stability in life. The family structure would dissolve. We would all be a bunch of selfish assholes jumping from person to person until we turn 80 and realize that we should've just worked harder to make our relationships work, instead of throwing our hands up and walking away when things get tough. The grass is not greener on the other side. The grass is greener where you water it.

Use your new level of attractiveness, energy, and self-worth as a guide for your wife's future behavior. The new theme is, *"This is the way things are going to be from now on."* You're going to lead. You're going to be awesome and attractive, and she is going to appreciate it and reciprocate. She's going to put the same effort into her own self-improvement and work on your marriage.

You're worth it and she's worth it.

The results will be sexy, fun and positive. Yes, it's going to be tough. Really tough. This is why they say, *"Relationships are hard work"*.

Again, that doesn't mean you are telling her, *"Fuck me, or I leave, woman!"* This means you are now acutely aware of what a dead bedroom signifies. It means the relationship was on its last legs.

You've done all YOU can to remedy the situation, now it's up to her to do the same. It takes two to tango.

About Pity Sex

After publishing the first edition of The Dead Bedroom Fix, some of the most commonly asked questions I received from readers revolved around the topic of "pity sex". "Pity sex" is what we call the sex that our wives offer us even though they are obviously not turned on. They do so out of obligation… or to just shut us up. For anyone who has a sense of empathy and smidgen of social awareness, you can spot "pity sex" a mile away.

Often, when a guy starts his journey of self-improvement, a wife will pick up on it right away.

First it starts as, *"Hmmm… something is weird here."* She will poke and prod and look for something insidious bubbling under the surface. When she fails at uncovering anything sinister, she's left with the realization: *"Oh, he's just getting better. He's getting more attractive. Now I'm kinda scared I may lose him and my entire comfortable existence may come to an end."* While this may be the beginning of the process of genuine attraction and appreciation, it's not the entire recipe you need to make the complete "wife is crazy about me" stew you're looking for.

Your wife: *"We can have sex tonight, if you want."* This can happen relatively quickly. After all, thanks to "women's intuition" they can pick up on changes in social dynamics fairly easily. She knows something is up, she knows it can lead to something really "wrong", so she does what she feels is the full-proof method for getting her husband back in line: She offers him sex.

My word of advice is this: You don't have to have sex if you don't want to. If your eyes and your gut are telling you, *"This doesn't' feel right"*, and you're sure that she's offering you sex for the wrong reasons, then politely decline. I think you should err on the side of complete honesty. *"Honey, you don't have to do that. I realize you FEEL like you have to, but you don't. Really. Your body language is all off. You don't look the least bit into it. I'd much prefer to wait until you're 100% comfortable and really in the mood. Okay? Honestly… no hard feelings at all. I get it completely. I love you, beautiful."*

Wow, your wife won't know what to think. She will be further anxious, concerned, confused… and she will respect the hell out of you. Why? Because you're a man who is not a slave to his balls. You're not some horny teen who grabs at the first opportunity for sex. You're a man who has the social intelligence and the heart to say, *"I see what's going on here… it's not good. No thank you."* This is the epitome of being the "Mentally Healthy Non-Needy Man" (MHNNM) I described earlier.

You want true passion and desire. Your wife does, too. Be the leader and show her what is acceptable and what isn't. Show her that you don't have to settle for scraps. You can wait until you have the full recipe and the delicious sex stew you deserve.

Don't Get Comfortable

Trust me, it will take NO time at all to wipe out all the hard work you put into making these positive changes. At times, it will seem like the whole world is conspiring to bring you down and squash all your positive results. There will be temptations around every corner. Awesome food to eat. Lazy Sundays with a stack of pancakes and a couch calling your name. Friends making fun of you for working out so much. Family worried that you seem to have lost so much weight. *"Are you ill? You're not eating enough!"*

What will astound you is that your WIFE will seem to be the one that's most eager to sabotage your efforts. That's right, the one person who benefits the most from your changes (other than yourself) will try her damndest to bring you down.

You think you've seen "tests" before? Well, just wait. You ain't seen nothing yet, amigo.

You're going to present her a new man that pushes her buttons and makes her sexual engine rev back up. This is huge. This is no minor occurrence. This throws everything off balance. Her hindbrain is going to be screaming, **"THIS IS AMAZING… BUT MAKE SURE HE IS FOR REAL!"**

You'll get little insults at strange times. You'll get complaints. She'll try to shame you out of going to the gym. She'll question why you're dressing so nicely. She'll get more jealous. She'll start getting angry again about you looking at that woman at the mall for a split second. She may even attempt to shame you for it.

You shouldn't care one little bit.

This is the time when a lot of guys fold… and then they have to start all over again. *"Well, I mean.. she IS giving me sex now, so maybe I should ease up a bit."*

Don't you dare change. You'll be back at your old life faster than you can say pornhub.com.

Watch what she does, not what she says.

Look at your wife's appearance. I bet it has improved. Sex has gone up. When she's not throwing random tests your way, she's brighter and more energetic. Her spark has returned.

Married life is overall better.

Recognize the intent and feeling behind these random tests from your wife. It's fear, not anger. It's insecurity. She's scared of losing you and she's also scared that she's letting her guard down for a man that is not genuine. She's afraid that she's trusting a fraud. Show her comfort by continuing to be the best man you can be. Show her love and appreciation. Continuing to improve. Don't put up with her bullshit… and bang her with the force of a thousand rabid hyenas.

Remember, with sex comes drama. With drama comes sex. It's all part of the game.

CHAPTER 7
It Didn't Work

"Failure is only the opportunity to begin again, and this time more wisely.'"

Henry Ford

I'm Not Going to Bullshit You. All Your Hard Work May Not Result in Sex from Your Wife.

Yes, that's right. You could very well become the absolute best version of yourself, stop doing the five mistakes, stop putting up with your wife's bullshit, be a more loving partner, be a great leader… and she may still have no interest in sex or any kind of intimacy with you.

So, what's going on here?

Well, it could be a variety of things. It could be something terrible, like she is seeing somebody else on the side and wrote you off long ago. It could be that she has a great deal of resentment towards you (possibly for very valid reasons) and she views all these improvements and changes as happening way too late in the game. It could be hormonal. Is she permimenopausal? Hormones can have dramatic effects on a person's sex drive. For many women, menopause means that they close the chapter on their sexuality for good.

It could be that she never really was into you sexually but viewed you only as a provider of resources she needed for her and her future kids.

Many times, a man at this stage in the game becomes clear-headed and has a great number of epiphanies about their marriage. The fog of their previous provider-centric role

179

has lifted, and they now see things from a more "complete" viewpoint. What was once a woman who he raised children and maintained a home with is now a very angry and cold person who hasn't shown him affection for years.

He has been married to a genuine, died-in-the-wool asshole. The more he thinks back on their time together, the worse his opinion of his wife gets.

Wives who are "over" their relationship typically don't just walk up to their husband and say, "We're done" (unless another man is in the picture). Instead, they will gradually plant seeds of disdain in the hopes that their man will take the not-so-subtle hints and get the ball rolling himself. This allows the women to save face and play victim, but still get out of the awful life-sucking relationship.

Win/Win for her.

What she doesn't know is that her man is so conditioned and so broken that he will just double down on his "positive" attributes (the five mistakes) and hope to turn things around.

Men use their sense of "honor" as a badge of courage, when it's really just an excuse to roll over, expose their belly and submit to a wife who is nothing short of disgusted by them. I've heard horror stories from men about wives who treat them with over-the-top disdain. One man caught his wife spitting into his drink when she thought he wasn't looking. Another found text messages from his wife to another man saying that she hopes her husband's cancer treatment doesn't work so that he can hurry up and die. Another man watched his wife make fun of his asthma to a group of friends… Rolling her eyes in disgust.

Women are human beings. They are capable of some pretty malevolent behavior. If they feel that they are pushed into a corner (like being trapped in a boring life with a man they have lost respect for), they will act out. They may build up resentment and no-holds-barred hatred for their husband and act accordingly.

So, why doesn't YOUR wife respond positively to anything YOU do?

Who knows? Who cares?

As you get to this point in your transformation, something should have clicked in your brain. I alluded to this in the previous chapter where I talked about the possibility that you may no longer have sexual desire for your wife.

You are only responsible for you. You are not responsible for the opinions and actions of others. Sometimes that is disappointing and incredibly heartbreaking. It's can also be extremely liberating.

You get to be what YOU want to be.

That is life in a nutshell.

Always remember one thing: Relationships, by their nature, are very difficult.

Anyone who tells you otherwise is either bullshitting you, somehow lucked into a perfect partnership, or they are just "naturals" at navigating the turbulent relationship waters. They may be one of the chosen few who make this whole game look easy.

Why do I say that relationships are so difficult? Well, this is up for debate, obviously, but I have come to one big conclusion after my experience with my own marriages, the stories from my thousands of readers, and the many hours of research and reading I have done on the subject:

Marriage, as we currently know it, is not for most of us.

Marriage takes a certain disposition, a certain personality, and a specific set of life and relationship skills that most of us just flat out do not have.

If you stop and look at the modern-day interpretation of marriage, it's damn near impossible to get it right. Those of us wanting to get married are saying:

I want to be married to my best friend.

I want to be married to a good earner. Going through life is tough. We need money. We need security.

I want to be married to somebody I admire. With no respect

means I don't stick around.

I want to be married to my lover. I want to have desire for them on a consistent basis, and vice-versa.

I want to be married to my caregiver. I may get ill or incapacitated, and I want my spouse to be there for me no matter what.

Basically, we're saying, *"I want to have all of my relationship needs put into one human being from now until the day I die. I want my friend, my parent and my sexual lover all wrapped into one person."*

Wow… that's a lot of pressure. That's quite the list of expectations.

No wonder it fails so often.

But man… when it works… it's a beautiful thing.

Is it worth all of your hard work? Are you up for the challenge? Well, unfortunately, you're just one half of the equation. She has to want it, too… and she may very well not see the need or have any desire to improve upon your current marital situation, no matter what you do.

It sucks, but it's extremely common. Your wife gave up on your marriage.

Don't feel too bad about yourself. This is not a time for a

pity party. You're desirable. The new you could get laid next week by a pretty woman who just wants to have fun with a guy exactly like you. Your wife still saying *"get away from me"* should NOT be a giant reality-shattering event. It's just a fork in the road of life. It's tough… but not unexpected and by no means life-ending. In fact, the fun has just begun, as you will quickly learn.

Good life lesson for you: Don't gauge your worth based on the fickle opinion of others. You've done too much hard work and too many good things up to this point to say, "If she doesn't like me, then there must still be something wrong with me."

Maybe there is. Maybe there isn't.

Who gives a shit?

You should be content with the fact that you did absolutely ALL you could do to save your marriage. You presented the absolute best "husband" package possible to your wife. You accepted the challenge that comes with being a married man and faced it head on. You worked hard. You did everything by the book.

1. You're objectively more attractive.
2. You're healthier.
3. You have more energy.
4. You have stronger boundaries and more confidence.
5. Other women find you attractive.
6. Men look up to you.

7. You've made your attraction to your wife and intent known.
8. You're a loving and attentive husband.

All these positives things occurred in your life as a result of your hard work, and yet your wife says, *"Meh... I don't think so."*

Well, that's her problem.

You're a damn good husband. You're a good man. Don't forget that. With or without your wife, you are still YOU.

The dead bedroom signifies that there are major issues with your relationship. You just tried all you can to reignite your love life. You have been rejected. Your romantic relationship is over.

It's time to leave your wife.

Surprised I would suggest ending the marriage? Remember what I said at the beginning of this book: "This book was written for heterosexual men in long-term monogamous relationships who want more sex. "

I didn't say, *"More sex from your wife"*.

You're a good-looking, confident, interesting, fit, manly, kind, and hard-working dude.

I promise you. You'll be more than fine.

Frequently Asked Questions & Comments

After writing the first edition of The Dead Bedroom Fix, I receive A LOT of emails from readers. Here are a few of the most common ones:

"I want to get away from the house more. You said in the book that the lover doesn't really tell the woman his whereabouts or what he is doing. I tried this and my wife flipped out and said it was not a good thing. She didn't know if I was alive or dead."

Well… the quintessential Lover also dates and has sex with several different women at once. I don't suggest that for a married man… much like I don't suggest you run off and not tell the wife where you're going. I wouldn't expect my wife to do that, either. It would be weird.

When you're a married man with kids, it's important that you strike a balance between Lover and Provider. In my opinion, just walking out the door of your house and not telling anyone where you are going is strange. There's nothing wrong with saying, "Heading out to get some things done. Be back in a couple of hours. I may hit the gym, too. I'll let you know." You're not just dating the woman casually. You're her husband and father to her children.

"Should I tell my wife about this book? She's already noticed my change in behavior and is suspicious."

In other words, you're scared that your wife may think

you're up to no good. You want to alleviate her anxiety. You want to prove to her that your actions are done in a positive way. No, don't tell her. Stay the course. You're doing nothing wrong. I repeat: You're doing nothing wrong. Stop looking for mommy's permission and stop trying to fix her perceived negative emotions over something silly like, "My husband is finally acting like a man. Something must be wrong."

"My wife says I've been nothing but a huge asshole since I read The DB Fix. Our sex life hasn't improved at all. The other day I was going out the door and she asked me where I was going. I just said 'Out'. She blew up my phone with angry text messages. I ignored her. She later asked me if there was something I was pissed about. I wanted to tell her, 'Yes. I'm pissed that we haven't had sex since our two-year-old was born', but I know that's exactly what I shouldn't do. We've had those talks fifty times already. It doesn't do anything. Not sure what to do. I just told her that no, nothing is wrong."

I think by simply saying, "Out", it came across as a pissy and angry. And rightfully so. You're pissy and angry. SHE KNOWS exactly what you're upset about (at least, in part). How do I know she knows? Because you're a man and you've had the dreaded talk fifty times already. It has obviously affected you a great deal, and you're letting her know that in a very passive-aggressive way. Either get over it, move on and try to better yourself (regardless of her feelings), or simply tell her that you're not happy with the way the relationship is going and you're trying to process

things and you wish to be alone instead of whining to her
like you always do.

"So, I read your book and was ready to start putting in the
hard work to become a better man, but my wife surprised
me by asking if I've ever thought about having an open
marriage. That was a shock, to say the least. What do you
think about open marriages? Good idea? Seems to be a
good solution to our situation."

I think your wife is cheating on you.

"My problem is that your book assumes that there
was a super sexual point early in the relationship. My
relationship with my wife has never been sexual. I've
always felt like a pervert for wanting to do sexy things with
her. She hates doing anything beyond missionary in the
dark.. and I get that maybe once a month if I'm lucky. After
our child was born, we went a year and a half without sex.
Not all relationships can be saved, I'm afraid."

You're absolutely right. Read chapter 7 again.

"I loved the book and I agree with everything you said,
but I really don't think this will work with my wife. We're
so far gone it's not even funny. I'm afraid I've started an
emotional affair with another woman and I'm to the point
where I don't even care if my wife finds out. What did she
expect? Am I wrong for having these needs?"

No, you're not wrong for having needs. You're not wrong

for lusting after another woman. You're wrong for not doing the adult thing and sitting down with your wife and telling her it's over. Instead, you're taking the chickenshit way out and fooling around with another woman. You don't want to disrupt the comfort and stability of home life, but you also want to have your kicks on the side. You wouldn't be the first man in history to have an affair, and you also won't be the first to have his life blow up when his wife finds out (and she will find out).

"I read The Dead Bedroom Fix, but I was disappointed. It was basically all about going to the gym. There's more to being a man than just muscles. Not all of us want to be meatheads."

I can't tell you how many times I've been told this. It always baffles me. The gym is literally step one of a multi-step process outlined in the book. Why do so many men stop there and shut the book in disgust? Well, they're looking into a giant mirror. Their glaring faults are staring right back at them. Nobody likes being told, "You have a glaring negative trait and it's all your fault." Nobody likes being told, "You have a lot of work to do and that may involve doing physical things that are BELOW your perceived value." Many PhD and higher education types bristle at the thought of their brainy wives being turned on by muscles. Many of these guys also learn the hard way that their multiple degrees and their splendid doctoral dissertation don't make their wives' panties fly off. Then, they get really upset when they catch her with the pool man who can barely string a coherent thought together.

The book is not all about the gym. Don't be ridiculous. You just got scared when you read the truth and you threw the book down in disgust.

"My marriage started falling apart due to money issues. I lost my job early on and had a really hard time finding a job. We had to live off of my wife's income for over a year. Now I'm back to making more than what I did before, but we're still paying off debt. Our sex life went into the toilet as soon as I lost my job, and it hasn't been back since. I don't think getting in shape and being more assertive will help my situation. I think my problem is a common one and I'm surprised it wasn't covered in the book."

Your marriage broke down because your wife's security was threatened. You could've accomplished the same thing by having an affair, having a secret drug habit, or something else that says to your wife, "Sorry, you didn't pick the right guy". Instead, you lost your job and didn't have a new one right away. You put her in the role as the breadwinner. No, that's not a not a good formula for marital happiness. Yes, money is a huge stressor for anyone… but I can't tell you how many men tell me a story very similar to yours… only to discover that his wife was having a torrid affair with some unemployed loser.

Just food for thought.

"I'm confused about the concept of 'shit tests'. I find that my wife is constantly making disrespectful remarks. I've been good about ignoring them, but yesterday she told me that

she can tell I'm pissed off and wants to know why."

There's a fine line between "typical wife shit test behavior" and "toxic disrespectful behavior that needs to be called out immediately". Context is everything.

If you're on your way to the gym and your wife says, "Do you HAVE to go? Couldn't you stay here instead? You're always going to the gym. I was hoping we could stay in and snuggle today", that is a shit test. She's seeing how committed you are to your mission. She wants to see what you're made of. This should not piss you off. This should show you that you're on the right path. She loves you.

If your wife says, "I don't know why you are going to the gym. You still look the same as you always have. I don't know who you're trying to impress. It's not like you're ever going to look good with your shirt off" she's being disrespectful. Of course this upsets you.

Here's a phrase I try to teach men to use when their wife is disrespectful and toxic: "Okay, why would you say that? I can't imagine ever talking to you that way. It's extremely disrespectful and I expect a lot better from you. Do you understand me?"

That's not needy. That's not feminine. That's not weak. That's being a strong guy who's not afraid to call out bad behavior when it happens. He can deal with the subsequent drama.

Reader Stories

I Ithought I would share some of the stories from readers of the first edition of The Dead Bedroom Fix. Do you have your own story to share? Please feel free to shoot me message at dso@dadstartingover.com. I try my best to read and reply to every email.

DSO,

Okay, this book was so much like my story that I thought you were spying on me. One thing that stuck out at me was the part where you talk about men discovering that their asexual wife was really slutty in her past. That was totally my story. After we had our kid, my wife shut down sex completely. At first we could only use hands on each other (still sore from the baby)... then we could just cuddle and make out... then we could only cuddle... then we could only hold hands. After I literally cried to her about our lack of sex (wow I was such a pussy), she told me that she thinks she may be asexual. She said she literally has no more sex drive, and she never really did. She said sex was never really important to her. I asked her if that meant she was faking it all the first couple of years of our relationship because she seemed to enjoy it quite a bit back then. She said yes, she thinks she was. She's not sure. That always confused me. How do you not know if you enjoyed sex?? Seems to be a pretty cut and dry thing to me.

Something in my gut said that my wife's comment about being asexual was really weird and wrong. I know she was sexual before. I know she had relationships before me. I remembered you saying something about women cheating being common, so I started spying on her (not my proudest moment). I didn't find an affair, but I did find a conversation with one of her friends that made my jaw drop. She admitted to her friend that she was really "experimental" when she was in her 20's and had two different threesomes. She said she loved every minute of it. She told her friend all the dirty details. It was like reading porn. Then she said the thing that really hit me. "I forget what it's like to be wanted and sexy. I don't feel like a woman anymore." WOW. No mention of me at all. Her friend didn't even ask. It was like I didn't exist. I was begging her for sex for YEARS. I was crushed. That was my lowest point. Like your book said, my wife wanted sex but just not with me.

I saw your book on my Instagram feed. I bought it and read it all on the same day. It hit me so hard that I vowed right then and there to change myself completely. If my "asexual" wife doesn't want me, then so be it. I'm only 38, so I'm literally in the prime of my life. I couldn't go on living like that. I was looking forward to my new life without her.

I lost 30 pounds in 4 months. I changed my wardrobe completely. I started being more of a leader at the office and at home. I stopped asking for sex. I was still loving and sweet when my wife deserved it but I never took it to the next level and asked her for sex. Never. I could tell that my wife was really confused. It was around month number three that she started to act flirty and sexy around me. That's when she started asking me if I was happy with us. I just told her that there was always room for improvement. I tried to avoid the conversation. I just kept busy and went out of the house. I would spend a lot of time at my friend's house helping him put together a new wood shop in his basement. We would *drink beers and talk while working. It was great. When I wasn't with my friend I was at the gym. When I was home I would do my part and help clean up and take care of the kids. I never made a move towards my wife. Ever.*

About a month after our talk my wife texted me a link to a video on Pornhub. She asked me if we could please do the things in the video. I had to pick my jaw up off the floor. I thought it was a joke or a test at first. I was actually kind of mad. I wanted to text her back, "What happened to you being ASEXUAL?!" I didn't reply right away. I decided to take things in the other direction. I played the dominant role and told her that I expected her to be completely nude and bent over for me in bed when I get home. And guess what… she did! Of all our years together, that was the absolute best sex we've ever had.

My wife tests me all the damn time now. I usually pass the tests. That's probably my least favorite part of this change. Constant testing. But, she's never been happier. We have sex at least three times a week now. What's funny is that now our sex is very dom/sub where I tell her what to do, she follows, and we use all kinds of toys. We even take the dom/sub arrangement outside of the bedroom. It's something that we've both really gotten into and learned a lot about. It's amazing.

Thanks so much for writing the book. You've literally saved my marriage and gave me the best sex life I could imagine.

R.

DSO,

Just wanted to send an email to say thanks for putting together some help for guys going through the rough times in their marriage.

I've taken what you've said on board and it's helped more than any counselling sessions I've been to.

As a result, my wife and I are more intimate and more playful which is really what my goal was. I find the difficult part now is not sliding back into the same mindset as before (which is where I screwed up) and becoming complacent.

Thanks for the help, mate. Cheers and keep up the great content.

D.

DSO,

My wife and I have been in marriage counseling for over a year. It was my idea. I was tired of zero love and affection from her. Zero sex. The good part about going to counseling is that we really open up and talk about everything. We both feel better and closer after the sessions. We hold each other more. Every time we go to the counselor, she asks about how things are in the bedroom. My wife refuses to say anything about it other than she is not ready... and I end up just taking over the session and telling her how much it hurts me. The counselor actually agreed with me that withholding intimacy is a passive aggressive way of her resenting me. She admits that she resents me but she doesn't ever agree to have sex. So we're at a standstill.

I saw your book on Facebook and bought it. Everything made sense. It finally all clicked. I went to the counselor with her again and said that I was tired of talking about things and that I'm going to work on me instead of US from now on. The counselor liked my thoughts and my "new energy" but my wife didn't. She was just more resentful and it seemed to set us back even more.

I told myself that I was giving your ideas three months before I went to an attorney to talk about divorce. By month number two my wife came into the shower with me one morning and gave me oral sex. She hasn't done that since we started dating. I couldn't believe it. That same night she put the kids to bed and then told me to go to the bedroom for a surprise. I was amazed. My first thought was that I really need to buy DSO a beer!

I asked my wife why her sudden change of heart. She said she finally felt like I wasn't just all about sex but instead about our marriage and becoming a better couple. I was shocked. I was actually more selfish than I've ever been and she saw it as me working on us. Wow. I will never understand women.

Thank you for all you do. You saved our marriage. Let's get together for that beer!

J.

DSO,

To make a very long story short, I was the perfect Nice Guy to my wife for ten years. The last five years or so, I'd say we have had sex probably ten times total. She has been obivously turned off completely by me, but swears it's not my fault she doesn't want to have sex.

I read your book, stopped making the mistakes, and this past month we've had more sex than the past five years total. Swear to God.

I was pretty angry at first. I've been told by her that I need to be nice and live by happy wife happy life, and she always secretly hated it. As soon as I grew a backbone she suddenly likes me again. Not sure why she didn't just tell me what she wanted but I also know that she's not a man so she won't do that. She'll just test me instead.

I hope everything keeps going in the same direction. After living like this I can't go back to the old me again.

Thanks for writing the book and showing up on my Facebook feed.

L.

DSO,

My story is probably not like the rest of them. I was in a sexless marriage for years. I read your book and it really hit home for me. I did everything wrong. You also made me realize that my gut may have been right all along and my wife was cheating on me. Looks like there were at least two guys she was seeing but probably more. We divorced and she robbed me blind. I do get to see the kids half the time so not all is lost.

There is good news though. I started dating and using what I learned from your book and the sex has been crazy. The girl I'm seeing now actually said to me that she's glad I'm a real man and can actually make a decision. She says all the other men she dated acted like girls. I just had to laugh. I used to be one of those guys.

Thank you for all your hard work.

F.

DSO,

I thought you might like this story. After our last coaching session I did what you said and decided to not be scared to talk and be a little flirty with other women in front of my wife. As you know, because of a previous huge drama moment we had early in our marriage, that was something I've always been scared of.

We had my company Christmas party last month. There's a very attractive single manager of the company that was being especially friendly to me. She's about ten years older than me, but could easily pass for younger. Drop dead gorgeous.

Every guy at the office talks about her. She's divorced. My wife has said before that she doesn't like her, which is code for her being jealous.

As you know our sex life has improved a great deal since I put into use the things I learned from you and the DB Fix. I still wanted to have that crazy sex life we had before we had kids. We came close, but my wife still seemed to be holding back and not letting her freak flag fly again.

Well, we went to the party and the attractive manager lady was there. After a few drinks that night she wouldn't leave me alone. She literally hung on to me all night. My coworkers though it was the funniest thing they ever saw. My wife sure didn't think so! She didn't make a scene, but you could tell that she was upset all night. On the drive home she said, "Your friend sure seems to like you an awful lot." I just smiled and said, "Well, I can't blame her." That was NOT something I would ever normally say. Old me would explain that she was ugly, she meant nothing, I only have eyes for my wife, she is crazy to even be a little jealous...

I'll skip the dirty details, but we had the best sex of our entire relationship that night. I still can't believe the things my wife was willing and able to do. Unfuckingbelieveable.

Thank you, DSO! I'm so glad I found your book and got the help from you I needed.

Q.

DSO,

Thanks so much for writing The DB Fix. That book was exactly what I needed for my marriage. My wife actually found the book on my iPad and got very upset. She cried and said she felt horrible for not wanting sex and she wishes she did. I just told her I understand her point and I'm done pressuring her to do something she doesn't want to do. I said I was doing the hard work for me, not for us. She was angry after that (she said it sounded like I wanted to divorce) and didn't talk to me for a week. I was actually pretty damn close to divorcing her at that point. I met with an attorney to see what it would cost me. Let's just say it wasn't good and I decided to give my marriage another chance. LOL.

It took probably three months until my wife woke up one morning crying and saying that she felt bad for how she's been treating me and she sees how hard I've been working on myself and our marriage. She tried to give me oral, and it took all of my energy to stop her. I told her I didn't want pity sex with a crying woman, I wanted a wife that really WANTS me and that I was hoping that would be her. She cried and begged me not to divorce her. She said if I didn't want sex then what else is there for her to do. I just told her that maybe she should put the same work into herself and our marriage like I have. She said I was right and that she would.

She was true to her word. She joined the same gym I go to. She stopped all junk food. She dresses sexier. She lost 49 pounds. She's happier around the house. She treats me with love instead of treating me like an annoying child. For the *first time in our marriage I feel like she's chasing and trying to impress me instead of the other way around.*

We started having sex again and it's been fantastic. Right now I have zero complaints about our marriage.

Thanks again for writing the book!

E.

From Facebook – Private Group for Men in Dead Bedrooms:

I thought I'd post an update tonight because there was something that was said that really stood out, which I'll get to.

Last night we were watching TV and she was nodding off. It got to be about 12:30 and she said she was going to lay down. So, I said yes me too, I have an early morning (gonna hit the gym early because they're finally open). We lay down in bed and chit chat for a bit while she's nodding in and out. She finally says,, "I'm going to fall asleep unless you're going to keep me up" I reply with "How am I going to keep you up?" (even though I know what she was getting at) she said "Oh, I don't know..." so I just said, "Yea, me either. I'm going to bed too. I have an early morning." I could have probably initiated things because she gave me the green light, but I knew it wasn't worth it because she was really tired and wasn't all there.

Fast forward to today. She made several sexual comments to me all day and told me how she wanted it the night before but she was just too tired. Then she proceeded to tell me she was fully rested tonight. So, obviously I just played everything smooth all day and didn't even act at all bothered by her.

Later on in the evening she started drinking some wine. We decided we were going to go out to a local pizza place and get some dinner. Kids didn't want to get off the Xbox to go so her and I just went. Refer back to the beginning when I said she said something that stood out. Well, on the way to dinner she says, "You know I really just think I needed you to be more of a lover to me to get me turned on and that's what you've been doing" then right after that she reaches over and unzips my pants and starts giving me road head. Holy fuck. LOL. She's never done that, not once.

Fast forward we eat dinner and the entire time all she's talking about is fucking. All I can think about is who the hell switched my wife out LOL. Well we get home and she takes the kids food upstairs and she comes downstairs and rips my pants off and starts going to town again. Next thing you know we're upstairs in the our bedroom and the rest is history. She's now sleeping like a baby lol.

At this point, I'm not even sure what I've done but I've just done basically what the book says to do in my own way and it's worked a damn miracle. That's 2 crazy weekends in a row. Sorry for the long post, just wanted to give an update and hopefully some encouragement for everyone to keep it up because this shit works.

M.

I'm really grateful & thankful for DSO's book randomly popping up on my FB feed one day. Without it, I really don't think I'd still be married for 18 years. I love my wife, but I was so frustrated with my marriage and lack of intimacy. Feeling rejected & unloved and most of all, unable to figure out why that was. That was the key. His book gave me simple, understandable reasons and unapologetic answers to why things weren't going well in my marriage. I'm a regular nice guy, so I need simple straight talk and I can't tell you how much better this easily readable book was so much more effective than the hundreds of hours spent in individual & couples counseling I did for years, and not to mention thousands of dollars cheaper. This book has made me a better man and has made my marriage much more fun, enjoyable and sexually satisfying...FOR BOTH OF US! She's more loving, playful, appreciative, supporting, affectionate, her mood is elevated, her attitude towards me is positive & affirming, and it's because I'm a better man. My only regret is that I didn't read it 10 years ago when things in my marriage started to change. I will always feel indebted to him for making a lasting impression on me and and making the life I wanted with my wife and kids.

J.

I was lost and thought I had tried everything. I think I googled something like dead bedroom and it lead me to the book. I read the reviews and couldn't wait to get my hands on it for myself. I implemented the rules and I can honestly say that I instantly starting seeing success. It has been a few months post dbf and I can genuinely say that we are the happiest we have ever been. I am stronger, more confident and over all content. The private group and fraternity are priceless and an endless source of support and information.

N.

I have a love/hate relationship with The Dead Bedroom Fix. I love it because it has changed the way I look at my relationship. Hate it because it was a kick in the nuts and made me admit my failures.

My behavior has changed towards her, and hers towards me.

I've implemented the changes, and see that although my bedroom seems dead, it's more on life support with signs of coming out of it because of what I have learned.

I pass most her shit tests, call her on her rejection BS with humor, notice more that needs to be done around the house and do it before she mentions it and without wanting accolades.

We're butting heads with leadership, with her acquiescing more (albeit small things) to me.

She's walking around naked more around me now that I've taken her off the pedestal and I'm treating her like a person.

I know it's going to be a long road, but thanks to The Dead Bedroom Fix, it'll be a smooth road.

J.

Just wanted to show my appreciation to the DSO for introducing me to the Dead Bedroom Fix and getting me into a community of recovering nice guys. Not to mention it was my gateway to other books like No More Mr. Nice Guy. The way it's changed my life over the past three months is really incredible. It hasn't just changed my sexual life with my wife, but it's also affected my daily happiness and assertiveness at work.

Thankful for all of the harsh truths and reality checks. Somehow just being subscribed to the DSO fraternity (have been for a month now) doesn't seem like contribution enough. Let me know if there's every anything I can help out.

A.

DSO's no-nonsense straight talk writing style is the swift kick in the ASS that men need!

Men have been lied to and not taught how to really keep intimacy alive. Society tells you to give her everything she wants, submit to her demands, solve all her problems, and exhibit inherently feminine behavior.

DSO debunks several generations of progressive myths and lies and realigns the reader with the animalistic, primal impulses and how it applies in the 21st century marriage or long term relationship.

My bedroom was not dead but it was not trending the right direction. I was being passive, agreeable, and needy. My demanding work and the stressors of life had beaten us both down. I was letting her lead.

I read the book and within 2 weeks I had excellent results. Fast forward 2 months later and I have not had this much sex since I was in my early twenties. This is the most impactful book I've read in the last decade. This is a must buy for all men who look to drastically improve not only their bedroom but their marriage.

Thank you DSO!

J.

I don't recall how I stumbled across the Men in Dead Bedrooms private chat group. I joined the group and read everyone's posts and comments for a month. The wife and I have been fighting the worst we ever have. I was insulting her and screaming at her all the time. She was ready to leave me and I was ready to leave her.

I ordered the book and read it in one night and what an eye-opener. This book made me realize what a bad husband and lover I had become and no wonder my wife didn't want to make love to me. I realized I needed to fix myself, so I started walking 6km every morning to clear my mind when I woke up. I upped it to 10km in the morning to push myself more and added another 3-5km in the afternoons. (It's 30-35 degrees Celsius during my walks so they are not a walk in the park so to speak.) I then work out for 30-45 minutes. Then in the afternoon start a project around the house and finish it, yard work, building a basketball court with the kids, painting the house, I took online anger management course, I read self-help and improvement books in the evenings. I talk to a counsellor once a week and bitch to them not my wife.

I'm 43 never walked, worked out or took care of myself. I'm now changing my diet to get that six pack I always wanted, I'm tanning an hour a day plus the walking is helping my tan. It's only been 2 weeks but I'm such a different person, I talk calmly to my kids and wife and when we don't agree I just say my point and that's it, no arguing no more discussion. My kids take turns joining me on my daily walks, they are enjoying their new found Dad, my confidence is getting way better. My wife is respecting me more and initiated love making session after a massage which she has never done that! It's only been 2 weeks of hard work but I'm seeing progress, yes it's going to take months to get my six pack and full confidence. Hopefully by then my wife is jumping me and the passion has been reignited. If not atleast I gave her the best possible me and I'll be fine going forward.

Thanks DSO for opening my eyes and helping me with that first giant step.

M.

Let me know what you think.

Shoot me an email at dso@dadstartingover.com. I would love to hear what you thought about this book, both good and bad.

THANK YOU for reading. I hope it gave you a sense of hope and strength and put you on the right path to being a better dude... and getting more ass than a toilet seat.

Rock on, brother.

D.S.O.
www.dadstartingover.com

Join The DSO Fraternity!

For $9.99 per month, you will get DSO Fraternity member only articles and audio, live Zoom meetings with DSO and fellow members, access to Private Facebook groups, and access to all current and future books by DSO in PDF and Audiobook format. You also get discounts on one-on-one meetings with DSO. A portion of your monthly fee goes to support The Movember Foundation to help fight prostate cancer, testicular cancer and mental health issues for men. Join other men on their journey to being better men!

dadstartingover.com/join

The Dead Bedroom Fix by D.S.O.

http://www.dadstartingover.com

Cover by D.S.O.

Made in the USA
Middletown, DE
24 July 2021

44740434R00121